THE COMPLETE GUIDE TO
TEACHING EXERCISE TO SPECIAL POPULATIONS

Morc Coulson

Note

Whilst every effort has been made to ensure that the content of this book is as technically accurate and as sound as possible, neither the author nor the publishers can accept responsibility for any injury or loss sustained as a result of the use of this material.

Published by A&C Black, an imprint of
Bloomsbury Publishing Plc
36 Soho Square
London W1D 3QY
www.acblack.com
www.bloomsbury.com

First edition 2011

ISBN 9781408133187

A CIP catalogue record for this book is available from the British Library.

Acknowledgements
Cover photograph © Getty Images
Inside photographs © Chris Heron with the exception of Figure 16.3, page 211 © Shutterstock, pages 32, 34, 38, 64 © Joanne Miller
Illustrations by David Gardner
Designed by James Watson

This book is produced using paper that is made from wood grown in managed, sustainable forests. It is natural, renewable and recyclable. The logging and manufacturing processes conform to the environmental regulations of the country of origin.

Typeset in 10.75pt on 14pt Adobe Caslon by Saxon Graphics Ltd, Derby

Printed and bound in the United Kingdom by Martins the Printers

//CONTENTS

FOREWORD

Physical activity, in particular sport, has been an important part of my life since I was very young. I have been fortunate in that I have always had a talent for boxing, and I have also had people around me from an early age who have helped to nurture this talent and continue to do so. Being physically fit is an important part of boxing and means that I can continue to make a career out of what I love doing. I also feel that I benefit in terms of psychological and emotional well-being as a result. I would therefore encourage anyone wanting to get involved in supervising physical activity to try to improve their knowledge so that they can help individuals from all walks of life to feel the benefit as I do. *The Complete Guide to Teaching Exercise to Special Populations* is an excellent book that can help either those with experience or those who are just starting out with practical and theoretical information relating to a host of conditions.

Tony Jeffries, Professional Boxer
Bronze medal 2008 Olympics. Professional fights: seven wins and one draw. Amateur fights: 95. England vests: 56. BBC North East Sports Personality of the Year 2008. Silver medal EU Amateur Championship 2008; Bronze medal EU Amateur Championship 2005; Bronze medal EU Amateur Championship 2004.

ACKNOWLEDGEMENTS

Just a quick thanks to all who helped out on the book, especially to Chris Heron who did the photographs and to my wife Lorretta who pointed out that men have thicker skin than women, which is why she is always cold!

Morc Coulson
2011

// INTRODUCTION

The main purpose of this book is to provide a practical resource for those people involved or wanting to be involved in the delivery of physical activity to those with specific health conditions, referred to as 'special populations'. This book is also useful for those individuals who have been identified as being in a special population category and who are interested in taking up some form of physical activity. This book is also designed to be used as a study guide to complement any training qualification, as the information provided here is based on up-to-date research and information provided by relevant professional bodies. There are some terms that are used throughout the book that might not be familiar to all readers. For example, the term 'physical activity' is used extensively to describe any form of movement, exercise or activity that increases energy expenditure. This can range from gym-type exercise to activities such as gardening and washing the car. Another term that might not be familiar is related to a unit of measurement used in some of the diagnostic tests within. This unit is a 'mmol', which means, in simple terms, a very small amount. For example, when measuring blood cholesterol, the units used are mmol per litre of blood (mmol/l).

SPECIAL POPULATIONS

There is no universally accepted definition of the term 'special population', but it is often meant as a collective term for a group of people with certain health-related conditions. The term possibly originates from the health and fitness industry and relates to training and qualifications required by fitness instructors for the purpose of delivering physical activity programmes to those that need certain consideration outside of the apparently 'healthy population' – in other words, those people with health-related conditions that are not covered in general fitness qualifications but are covered on specific training courses designed for these conditions. The National Quality Assurance Framework, which was set up by the Department of Health in 2001, states that the minimum level of qualification recommended for exercise professionals who are responsible for designing and delivering physical activity programmes for low-to-medium risk referred patients, is a level 3 advanced instructor award with a recognised exercise referral qualification. Exercise referral is the general term that relates to a scheme that is normally run by a GP's (doctor's) surgery or medical centre whereby people with certain

Medical approval and qualification recommendations for all conditions

Condition	Medical approval		Specific qualification	
	Essential	*Recommended*	*Essential*	*Recommended*
Obesity		✓ (to identify any related condition)	✓ (L4)	
Diabetes	✓ (type 1)	✓ (type 2)	✓ (L4)	
COPD	✓			✓ (L3)
Asthma		✓		✓ (L3)
Hypertension	✓			✓ (L3)
Hyperlipidaemia		✓		✓ (L3)
Arthritis		✓		✓ (L3)
Osteoporosis		✓		✓ (L3)
Parkinson's		✓		✓ (L3)
Multiple sclerosis	✓			P (L3)
CVD	✓		✓ (BACR)	
Stroke	✓		✓ (BACR)	
Younger age				✓ (L2)
Older age				✓ (L2)
Disability		✓		✓ (L2)
Ante- and postnatal		✓ (if currently inactive)	✓ (L2)	

Notes:
L2 = level 2 instructor award
L3 = level 3 advanced instructor award
L4 = level 4 specialist instructor award
BACR = British Association of Cardiac Rehabilitation (see chapter 12)

diagnosed conditions are assessed and given an individual physical activity programme, which is delivered by those who are qualified to do so (typically as part of an NHS-funded team). Those individuals on exercise referral schemes can, however, be referred in different ways. First, a visit to the GP might result in the diagnosis of a condition that requires admission to the scheme. On the other hand, individuals might be referred to the GP by some other mechanism. For example, those wishing to supervise a physical activity programme for an individual should always carry out some kind of screening to identify if the individual doing the activity is 'apparently healthy' or not. One of the most common forms used to do this is the Physical Activity Readiness

Questionnaire (PAR-Q) as can be seen in appendix 1 at the end of this chapter. Developed by the Canadian Society for Exercise Physiology, the PAR-Q is a short questionnaire that can help to identify possible risk factors for cardiovascular, pulmonary and metabolic disease. If no risk factors are identified (all questions answered 'no'), the form then encourages a programme of *low-to-moderate* physical activity to be undertaken relative to the fitness level of the individual. If any factors are identified (by the individual answering 'yes' to one of the questions on the PAR-Q), the form advises that they be referred to a GP prior to undertaking a programme of physical activity. The individual will then be assessed as to their suitability for an exercise referral programme, although the range of conditions that are accepted varies from surgery to surgery. The range of conditions within this book is designed to be comprehensive, in order to cover a wide spectrum of groups – from those who require limited medical intervention, such as the younger age group, to those who require a great deal of medical intervention, such as sufferers of cardiovascular disease. In order to help the reader, the table opposite presents an overview of the conditions for which medical approval is considered by the author to be an essential prerequisite, and those for which it is just a recommendation. The table also gives an overview of those conditions for which specific qualifications are considered by the author to be essential for those supervising activity, or whether these are just recommended. There are many training courses that deliver qualifications relevant to the conditions covered in this book, however the availability of courses for some of the conditions can be limited, and for others do not yet exist.

Information relating to available training courses, and the structure of qualifications and standards (known as National Occupational Standards) for the health and fitness industry is available from Skills Active (www.skillsactive.com), which is the sector skills council for active leisure in the UK. There is also a body known as the Register of Exercise Professionals (www.exerciseregister.org.uk), which provides information related to the levels of awards and how to register as part of the professional body.

ABOUT THIS BOOK

The book is organised into four distinct parts. First, chapter 1 deals with the relationship between physical activity and health, and the risks associated with low levels of physical activity (known as sedentariness or inactivity). It also looks at recommended guidelines and the numbers of people in the UK who follow them. The second part (chapters 2–13) covers those special populations for which there is only a potential risk of developing the particular condition and, in some cases, where physical activity substantially reduces that risk. The 'special populations' covered in these chapters are obesity, diabetes mellitus, chronic obstructive pulmonary disease (COPD), asthma, hypertension, hyperlipidaemia, arthritis, osteoporosis, Parkinson's disease, multiple sclerosis, cardiovascular disease (CVD) and stroke. Each chapter follows a typical layout, with sections as follows.

WHAT IS IT?

Each chapter starts with a description of the relevant condition. Some of the descriptions are more in depth than others, but this is not representative of how important each condition is thought to be, as all conditions within this book are considered to be of equal importance.

PREVALENCE

This simply refers to how many people are thought or estimated to have the condition. The author can rely only on research available at the time of this book's publication, and indeed the quality of that research. The very nature of some of the conditions makes it difficult for accurate figures to be acquired. Also, depending on the source of the research, some conditions will have global estimates, while others will have estimates only from the UK.

SYMPTOMS

Chapters 2–13 deal with a range of symptoms that are related to the specific condition. It should be understood, however, that symptoms do not always appear and in some cases there may be multiple symptoms, whereas in others there might be only one or two.

RISK FACTORS

All of the conditions described in chapters 2–13 have a range of factors (these can be related to lifestyle or have a genetic link) that are known as 'risk factors'. These are simply factors that increase the chances of a person developing the specific condition. It must be stressed that even if people have any of these factors, it is considered only a risk and not a guarantee that they will develop the associated condition. For example, those with high cholesterol levels do not always develop heart disease and those with high blood pressure do not always suffer a stroke.

DIAGNOSIS

There is a range of diagnostic tests associated with each condition. Some tests can be carried out only in a clinical environment by suitably qualified people, but some can be done outside of a clinical environment. In some of the chapters there are 'test boxes', which describe tests that can be done outside of a clinical environment as they are not designed as diagnostic tests. They are simply used to establish at what level the individual with the condition may be at in relation to the test so that the test can then be repeated at a later date to see if any improvement has been made. As there are contraindications to testing people with various conditions it is always advisable to consult a GP or specialist before undertaking any testing, and to have the individual complete an 'informed consent' or 'freedom of consent' form prior to any testing (see appendix 2 at the end of this chapter).

PHYSICAL ACTIVITY BENEFITS

Some of the conditions presented in this book are covered by a wealth of information relating to the benefits of physical activity, whereas others have only a limited amount. This is partly due to the problems associated with researching the particular condition. This part of the chapter tries to distinguish between the benefits of cardiovascular-type activity and resistance-type activity.

PHYSICAL ACTIVITY GUIDELINES

This part of the chapter tries to give general guidelines for both cardiovascular- and resistance-type activity in relation to type, frequency, intensity and duration. The section also presents information that has been taken from a variety of sources relating to associated precautions. Some conditions have very specific guidelines that are commonly agreed upon by professional bodies, whereas for other conditions the guidelines are more general and there are possible differences between sources. The activity guidelines within this part of the chapter recommend at what intensity the person should carry out the cardiovascular and resistance activities. This book refers to two different methods of setting cardiovascular intensity: percentage of maximum heart rate (%HRmax) and rate of perceived exertion (RPE). It also uses repetition maximum (RM) for setting resistance intensity. All methods are explained in appendix 3 and 4 at the end of this chapter.

The next part of the book (chapters 14–17) deals with those special populations for which physical activity does not reduce the risk as they are considered an actual consequence of life. The special populations covered in these chapters are younger age, older age, ante- and postnatal, and disabled people. The final part of the book is chapter 18, which offers an overview of medications related to the various special populations. This particular section is not meant to be a definitive guide but more of a quick reference, as information relating to conditions and medication changes very regularly. This section does however attempt to provide the reader with an understanding of the side effects related to specific medications that might be useful in relation to physical activity.

APPENDIX 1: PHYSICAL ACTIVITY READINESS QUESTIONNAIRE (PAR-Q)

Please read the following questions and answer each one honestly.

	Yes	No
Has your doctor ever said that you have a heart condition and that you should only do physical activity recommended by a doctor?	—	—
Do you feel pain in your chest when you do physical activity?	—	—
In the past month, have you had chest pain while you were not doing physical activity?	—	—
Do you lose your balance because of dizziness or do you ever lose consciousness?	—	—
Do you have a bone or joint problem that could be made worse by physical activity?	—	—
Is your doctor currently prescribing drugs for your blood pressure or heart condition?	—	—
Do you know of any other reason why you should not do physical activity?	—	—

If you answered YES to one or more questions

Talk to your doctor **BEFORE** you become more physically active or have a fitness appraisal. Discuss with your doctor which kinds of activities you wish to participate in.

If you answered NO to all questions

If you answered no to all questions you can be reasonably sure that you can:

Start becoming much more physically active – start slow and build up.

Take part in a fitness appraisal – this is a good way to determine your basic fitness level. It is recommended that you have your blood pressure evaluated.

However, delay becoming more active if:

You are not feeling well because of temporary illness such as a cold or flu.

If you are or may be pregnant – talk to your doctor first.

Please note: *If your health changes so that you then answer YES to any of the above questions, tell your fitness or health professional. Ask whether you should change your physical activity plan.*

'I have read, understood and completed this questionnaire. Any questions I had were answered to my full satisfaction.'

Name _____

Signature _____   Date _____

Signature of parent _____   Witness _____
or guardian

Note: This physical activity clearance is valid for a maximum of 12 months from the date it is completed and becomes invalid if your condition changes so that you would answer YES to any of the seven questions.

Source: Physical Activity Readiness Questionnaire (PAR-Q) 2002. Reprinted with permission from the Canadian Society for Exercise Physiology.

APPENDIX 2: TYPICAL INFORMED CONSENT FORM

In order to assess cardiovascular function, body composition, and other physical fitness components, the undersigned hereby voluntarily consents to engage in one or more of the following tests (check the appropriate boxes):

☐ Aerobic capacity test   ☐ Muscular strength tests

☐ Underwater weighing   ☐ Flexibility tests

EXPLANATION OF THE TESTS

The aerobic capacity test is performed on a bicycle or treadmill. The intensity is increased every few minutes for a period of 15 minutes. We or you may stop the test at any time because of fatigue or discomfort. The underwater weighing procedure involves being completely submerged in a tank or tub while breathing through respiratory equipment. This test provides an accurate assessment of your body composition. For muscular strength testing, you lift weights for a number of repetitions using free weights or exercise machines. These tests assess the strength of the major muscle groups in the body. For evaluation of flexibility, you perform a number of stretching-type exercises during which we measure the range of motion in your joints.

RISKS AND DISCOMFORTS

During the aerobic capacity test, certain changes may occur. These changes include abnormal blood pressure responses, fainting, irregularities in heartbeat and heart attack. Every effort is made to minimise these occurrences. Emergency equipment and trained personnel are available to deal with these situations if they occur. You may experience some discomfort during the underwater weighing, especially if you are fearful of being submerged. Breathing through respiratory equipment while underwater should minimise this discomfort. If necessary, alternative tests can be used to estimate body composition. There is a slight possibility of muscle strain or spraining a ligament during the muscular strength and flexibility testing. In addition, you may experience muscle soreness 24 to 48 hours after testing. These risks can be minimised by performing warm-up exercises prior to taking the tests. If muscle soreness occurs, appropriate stretching exercises to relieve this will be demonstrated.

EXPECTED BENEFITS FROM TESTING

These tests allow us to assess your physical working capacity and to appraise your physical fitness status. The results are used to help prescribe a safe and individualised exercise programme for you. Records of the tests are kept strictly confidential.

INQUIRIES

Questions about the procedures used in the physical fitness tests are encouraged. If you have any questions or need additional information, please ask us to explain further.

FREEDOM OF CONSENT

Your permission to perform these physical fitness tests is strictly voluntary. You are free to deny consent if you so desire.

I have read this form carefully and I fully understand the test procedures. I consent to participate in these tests.

Signature of participant .... Date ....

APPENDIX 3: PERCENTAGE OF MAXIMUM HEART RATE (%HRMAX)

One of the most common methods used to measure cardiovascular intensity is percentage of maximum heart rate (%HRmax). For example, if the individual has a goal of developing aerobic fitness, it would be recommended that they exercise at a heart rate level of between 70 and 80% of their maximum (the aerobic zone). This can be written as 70–80%HRmax. To use this method the maximum heart rate of the person is needed. As an actual maximum heart rate test is not recommended for the majority of the population, this needs to be estimated. There are many ways to estimate maximum heart rate but one of the easiest is to use the following formula:

Estimated maximum heart rate = 220 – age

The unit that heart rate is measured in is beats per minute (which is written as bpm). Once maximum heart rate has been estimated by using the '220 – age' formula, you then need to work out the recommended percentage for the particular individual. For example, in the chapter on obesity, cardiovascular activity is recommended to be performed at between 40 and 85% of maximum heart rate. If the individual who is to do the activity is 20 years old then the following steps should be used to work out their heart rate range.

Example
20 year old exercising between 40 and 85%HRmax

Step 1
Estimated maximum heart rate is 220 – age (20 years) = 200 bpm

Step 2
40% of maximum heart rate =
(200 ÷ 100 then × 40) = 80 bpm
85% of maximum heart rate =
(200 ÷ 100 then × 85) = 170 bpm

From this example it can be seen that the heart rate of a 20-year-old individual exercising at between 40 and 85% of maximum heart rate should be 80–170 bpm. This obviously has its problems as not everyone has access to or knows how to use heart rate monitors. Also, most people find it difficult to check their own heart rate, especially when exercising. For this reason an alternative method for setting intensity is that of rate of perceived exertion (RPE) (see appendix 4).

APPENDIX 4: RATE OF PERCEIVED EXERTION (RPE)

This particular method was designed many years ago by Dr Gunnar Borg and is essentially a scale relating to how people feel during activity. As can be seen in the accompanying table, there are two scales: the 6–20 and the 0–10 versions. Both are still used, even though the 0–10 scale is the later version. For the purposes of this book, the 6–20 scale will be used as it is often easier to use with lower intensities of activity.

Borg RPE scales		
6–20 scale	**0–10 scale**	**Estimate of %HRmax**
6	0 Nothing at all	
7 Very, very light	0.3 Practically nothing	
8	0.5 Extremely weak	50%
9 Very light	0.7	55%
10	1 Very weak	60%
11 Fairly light	1.5	65%
12	2 Weak	70%
13 Somewhat hard	2.5	75%
14	3 Moderate	80%
15 Hard	4	85%
16	5 Strong	88%
17 Very hard	6	92%
18	7 Very strong	96%
19 Very, very hard	8	98%
20	9	100%
	10 Extremely strong	
	11	
	Absolute maximum	

Source: Adapted from American College of Sports Medicine (2009) *ACSM Guidelines for Exercise Testing and Prescription* (8th edition), London: Lippincott Williams & Wilkins.

It can be seen that each scale relates to an approximate level of maximum heart rate, which makes it simple to use. For instance, in the example shown on page 10 of an individual being asked to work at between 40 and 85% of maximum heart rate, if the RPE scale is used they would be asked to work at between 7 and 15 on the 6–20 scale – in other words, between very, very light and hard. With this method there are no problems such as those that can be encountered with heart rate monitoring.

APPENDIX 5: REPETITION MAXIMUM (RM)

When prescribing a particular intensity of a resistance exercise for an individual (how heavy the weight should be), the intensity can be prescribed by using a multiple of the maximum capability of that individual. For example, the maximum weight that an individual is capable of lifting once is known as 1 repetition maximum (1RM). It follows therefore that a weight an individual can lift 10 times (but will fail on the 11th attempt) is known as 10 repetition maximum, or 10RM. Many guidelines that are written often just state the number of repetitions, such as 10–15 reps. In most cases this means 10–15RM or the maximum amount of weight that can be lifted between 10 and 15 times but no more. Repetition maximum can also be compared to the percentage of the maximum that a person can lift. For example, in the accompanying table, if an individual were able to lift a weight five times but would fail on the sixth attempt (5RM) they would be lifting approximately 86% of their maximum capability. Care must be taken, however, with those who are not familiar with this method. A period of practice – finding out just how hard this method can be – is very much recommended.

RM compared to percentage of maximum	
Repetition max	**% of max**
1	100
2	93.5
3	91
4	88.5
5	86
6	83.5
7	81
8	78.5
9	76

PHYSICAL ACTIVITY AND HEALTH

1

KEYPOINTS

- There are many potential health benefits from being active, including a lower risk of coronary heart disease, stroke, type 2 diabetes and certain types of cancer.
- Activity levels in England are low. About 60% of men and 72% of women report less than 30 minutes' moderate-intensity activity a day on at least five days per week.
- About 70% of boys and 60% of girls aged 2–15 achieve at least 60 minutes' physical activity each day of the week. However, 30% of boys and 40% of girls do less than 30 minutes' activity per day.
- Those people with a lower income are more likely to have low activity levels than those with a higher income.
- The cost of physical inactivity in England (costs of treatment and the indirect costs caused through work absence) has been estimated at more than £10 billion a year.
- Higher risks occur mainly with vigorous levels or contact sports and high-volume fitness training.
- Adults with low physical activity levels are more than twice as likely to have a raised waist circumference as those with high levels of physical activity.
- The health benefits of activity far outweigh the risks.
- Many recognised guidelines suggest that 30 minutes is the minimum amount of time a person should spend doing moderate-intensity activity each day.

ACTIVITY LEVELS IN THE UK

It is widely agreed that there are many health benefits of a physically active lifestyle and there is a large amount of research-based evidence to show that regular physical activity can help to reduce, by up to 50%, the incidence of many chronic conditions that occur as a result of sedentary behaviour. This is very important, not just from a health point of view, but also when it is considered that the cost to the nation as a result is more than £10 billion a year. Generally speaking, physical activity or exercise guidelines for adults normally recommend a minimum of 30 minutes of at least moderate-

Table 1.1	Description of low, medium and high physical activity levels
Activity levels	**Description**
Low	Active at a lower level or not active at all
Medium	30 minutes or more of moderate-intensity physical activity on 1 to 4 days in the last week
High	30 minutes or more of moderate-intensity physical activity on at least 5 days in the last week

intensity physical activity (such as brisk walking, cycling or climbing the stairs) on at least five days a week, which can be built up in bouts of 10 minutes or more throughout the day. The *Health Survey for England* report of 2008 that showed how physical activity guidelines (at different levels) for adults and children were being met between 1997 and 2006. In terms of the different levels, table 1.1 shows how low, medium and high physical activity levels were classified for the report.

The *Health Survey for England* report investigated physical activity levels among adults and children of both genders in England, and showed that the proportion of those achieving a minimum of 30 minutes of at least moderate-intensity physical activity at least five days a week had increased from 32% in 1997 to 40% in 2006 for men, and for women increased from 21% to 28% (fig 1.1 helps to illustrate this). The report also revealed a vast difference between adults and children, as about 70% of boys and 60% of girls aged 2–15 years achieved at least 60 minutes of physical activity each day of the week. In other words, almost twice as many children as adults are achieving the recommended guidelines for physical activity.

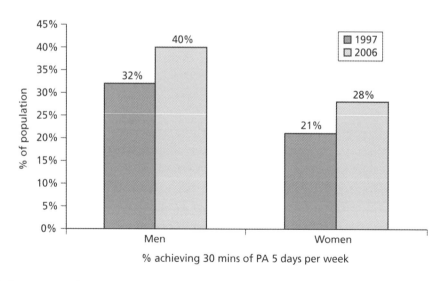

Figure 1.1 Percentage of male and female adults achieving specific physical activity (PA) guidelines

Table 1.2 Reported activities of adults from 2005 to 2007

Type of activity	Percentages	
	2005/6	2006/7
Swimming or diving (indoors)	15.7	14.5
Health, fitness, gym	13.8	13.8
Cycling (health, recreation, training or competition)	9.7	10.0
Snooker, pool, billiards	8.0	7.7
Football, including 5-a-side (outdoors)	7.0	7.6
Keep-fit, aerobics, dance exercise	6.9	6.8
Golf, pitch and putt, putting	5.6	5.5
Jogging, cross-country, road running	5.1	6.2
Swimming or diving (outdoors)	4.0	3.4
Tenpin bowling	3.6	3.7

Even though there were overall increases over the years in people achieving the minimum physical activity guidelines, there was a significant drop for those aged 75 years and over and it is still widely agreed that the great majority of adults in England do not participate in physical activity at levels that provide the full range of health benefits. The report also covered the type of activities that people took part in. For instance, in 2006 a higher proportion of both men and women reported participating in walking, and in sports and exercise, compared to 1998. For men, 32% reported walking briskly in 1998 compared with 38% in 2006. Likewise, reported participation in sports and exercise has risen for men from 42% to 46%. For women, 24% reported walking briskly in 1998 compared with 30% in 2006, while 36% participated in sports and exercise in 1998 compared with 39% in 2006. In 2009, the National Survey of Culture also published a report, which looked at the activities that adults in England took part in between 2005/6 and 2006/7. This was called the *Taking Part Survey*; it asked adults which activities they had participated in at least once in the previous four weeks. Of these activities, participation in outdoor football and jogging, cross-country and road running all increased, while participation in swimming, both indoors and outdoors, decreased from 2005/6 to 2006/7, as can be seen in table 1.2.

One of the main problems due to lack of physical activity is that of obesity levels. For instance, the *Health Survey for England* (2006) reported that physical activity levels were related to body mass index (BMI) and waist circumference, as both men and women with low activity levels were more likely to have a higher BMI and raised waist circumference (see chapter 2) compared to those with high activity levels. An interesting question in the 2006 survey was related to the government's guidelines for physical activity. In answer to this question, only 27% of men and 29% of women aged 16 to 64 years thought they knew the physical activity recommendations, and the majority of adults thought they were fairly active, even though more than two-thirds of adults said

Table 1.3	Physical activity targets for the UK in 2004*
Country	**Government target**
England	
Adults	By 2020, 70% of individuals to be undertaking 30 minutes of physical activity on at least 5 days a week (50% of individuals by 2011)
Children	Increase the proportion of school children in England who spend a minimum of 2 hours each week on high-quality sport from 25% in 2002, to 75% by 2006 and 85% by 2008
Wales	
Older people	To reduce the age-standardised rate for stroke mortality by 20% in 65 to 74 year olds by 2012 and at the same time narrow the gap between the most deprived and least deprived groups
Scotland	
Adults	To increase the proportion of all adults aged over 16 years taking the minimum recommended levels of physical activity (30 minutes of moderate activity on 5 or more occasions each week) to 50% by 2022; this means an average increase of 1% a year across the population
Children	To increase the proportion of all children aged 16 and under taking the minimum recommended levels of physical activity (1 hour a day of moderate activity on 5 or more days a week) to 80% by 2022; again, this means an average increase of 1% a year across the population

* There is no target for Ireland

they would like to do more physical activity, but barriers such as work commitments and lack of leisure time prevented them from doing so. For this reason, the easiest forms of physical activity that can be incorporated into everyday life – such as walking, cycling, gardening and social sporting activities – should be encouraged. Because of the concern relating to figures such as these, a target for physical activity in England, Wales and Scotland was proposed in 2004 by the Government's Strategy Unit (see table 1.3). This is a very ambitious target, however, considering that participation levels of adults in England would need to more than double in just over 15 years.

HEALTH RISKS OF PHYSICAL INACTIVITY

In 2002, a report from the World Health Organization (WHO) stated that physical inactivity is one of the ten leading causes of death in developed countries, resulting in more than 1.9 million deaths worldwide per year. *The World Health Report*, as it was called, estimated that around 3% of all disease burden in developed countries is caused by physical inactivity, and that over 20% of coronary heart disease (CHD) and 10% of stroke in developed countries is due to physical inactivity (stated by the report as less than 2.5 hours per week moderate-intensity activity or 1 hour per week of vigorous activity). There are many published reports that discuss the range of health risks associated with physical inactivity (or being sedentary, as it is usually referred to). As it would be difficult to discuss the whole range of publications, the following are an example of just some of the associated risks of being sedentary that commonly appear in many of the reports:

- coronary heart disease (CHD)
- stroke
- certain cancers
- diabetes
- hypertension
- osteoporosis
- obesity
- anxiety and depression
- osteoarthritis
- brain function
- painful conditions.

CORONARY HEART DISEASE (CHD)

It has been shown that in the UK about 38% of CHD-related deaths are as a result of physical inactivity or sedentary lifestyles. CHD accounts for around 24% of premature deaths in men and around 14% of premature deaths in women in the UK.

STROKE

It has been widely reported that stroke (see chapter 13) is already the second leading cause of death in the western world after heart disease, and is thought to be responsible for around 10% of deaths worldwide (an estimated 16 million first-time stroke patients and 5.7 million stroke deaths). Research suggests that moderately active people are less likely to have a stroke or die of stroke-related causes than those with low activity levels.

CANCER

Colorectal cancer accounts for about 3% of all premature deaths in both men and women. It is estimated that more than 7000 women in England alone died prematurely from breast cancer in the year 2000. It has been widely reported that regular physical activity is associated with a decreased risk of developing colon cancer, by up to 50%.

DIABETES

According to various sources, more than 1.5 million people in the UK have been diagnosed with type 2 diabetes. It is generally accepted that regular physical activity lowers the risk of developing non-insulin-dependent diabetes mellitus by as much as 50%. Risk may also be reduced in groups of people with impaired glucose tolerance (see chapter 3).

HYPERTENSION

According to the *Health Survey for England* in 2003, high blood pressure affects more than 16 million people in the UK and is the direct cause of about half of all strokes and heart attacks in the country. As a consequence, high blood pressure has resulted in about 62,000 unnecessary deaths every year. It is widely understood that regular physical activity prevents or delays the development of high blood pressure, and can also help to reduce systolic and diastolic blood pressure by up to 10 mmHg (see chapter 6).

OSTEOPOROSIS

It is estimated that around one in three women and one in twelve men in the UK over the age of 50 years will sustain a spine, hip or wrist fracture as a direct result of having osteoporosis. It is also estimated that about one in three of over-65s and about 50% of over-85s fall each year. Therefore, regular weight-bearing physical activity is essential for helping normal skeletal development. Strength training and other forms of exercise in older women have been shown to reduce the risk of hip fracture by up to 50% (see chapter 9).

OBESITY

In 2009 the National Health Service Information Centre published a report which stated that 24% of all adults were classified as obese in England in 2007, and that 65% of men and 56% of women were overweight in the same year (this is including those that are obese). It is well known that regular physical activity can reduce the risk of individuals becoming obese by as much as 50% compared to people with sedentary lifestyles (see chapter 2).

ANXIETY AND DEPRESSION

The psychological effects of anxiety and depression are very common in the UK, but can be difficult to measure as there are many people who suffer the effects but never seek help or advice. As there are many different effects linked to anxiety and depression, the research is varied but, generally speaking, regular physical activity appears to:

- relieve symptoms of depression and anxiety,
- improve mood and self-esteem and
- protect against the development of mild forms of depression.

OSTEOARTHRITIS

The National Institute of Arthritis and Musculoskeletal and Skin Diseases reports that osteoarthritis is more common in men before the age of 45 years and more common in women after the age of 45 years. The Institute also states that the condition is more prevalent in older age. Research has shown that an absence of stress on the joints can increase the risk of osteoarthritis (as can an excess of stress).

BRAIN (COGNITIVE) FUNCTION

As a rough estimate, in the UK there are about 18,500 people under the age of 65 years with dementia. It is thought that regular physical activity enhances and protects brain function.

PAINFUL CONDITIONS

There are numerous painful conditions that exist that can be positively affected by regular physical activity. Some of the common benefits of maintaining a regular programme of exercise include:

- helping to maintain the health of joints,
- controlling the symptoms of arthritis and osteoporosis,
- helping to improve stamina in people with disabilities,
- helping to prevent lower back pain and
- helping to manage lower back and knee pain.

As there are so many conditions that can be affected by physical activity (or inactivity), the volume of research that has been done over the years is vast and almost impossible to summarise. However, in 2004 the Department of Health published a report that included a summary of a

Table 1.4	Summary of evidence of physical activity effects on certain conditions	
Condition	**Evidence (low/medium/high)**	**Preventative effect (weak/moderate/strong)**
Coronary heart disease	High	Strong
Stroke		
– Occlusive	High	Moderate
– Haemorrhagic	Medium	Weak
Peripheral vascular disease	No data	
Obesity and overweight	Medium	Moderate
Type 2 diabetes	High	Strong
Osteoporosis	High	Strong
Osteoarthritis	No data	
Low back pain	Medium	Weak
Depression	Low	Weak
Mental function	Low	Moderate
Cancer		
– Overall	Medium	Moderate
– Colon	High	Strong
– Rectal	Medium	No effect
– Breast	High	Moderate
– Lung	Low	Moderate
– Prostate	Medium	Equivocal
– Endometrial	Low	Weak

review undertaken relating to the effect of physical activity on certain conditions. Table 1.4 provides a simplified summary adapted from the report, which shows the quality and strength of the available research evidence related to a particular condition. The level of evidence (high, medium or low) is intended to offer a general indication of the volume and quality of the available evidence. The table also estimates the strength of the preventative effect that physical activity can potentially have on the condition.

As can be seen, there are many health-related reasons for all individuals to include some kind of physical activity in their regular daily routine. One important statistic reported by the Department of Health in 2004 that can help reinforce this message is that active people have a 20–30% reduced risk of dying prematurely as inactive people. They also state that inactive people are almost twice as likely to have a heart attack as active people. For information purposes, the Department of Health classifies active people as having an energy expenditure of 500 to 1000 kcals per week, which is about 6 to 12 miles of walking (roughly 10,000 to 20,000 steps per week) for an average-weight individual. However, it should be highlighted that physical activity is not a 'quick fix' and that a lifelong approach to physical activity is necessary as sedentary behaviour, or inactivity, can have different detrimental effects throughout life. For example, health-related problems as a result of inactivity can begin in childhood, but it is often not until middle or even older age that these problems result in various conditions and even lead to premature mortality (death).

RISKS OF PHYSICAL ACTIVITY

Although the benefits of regular physical activity far outweigh the negative or detrimental aspects, it should be pointed out that there are certain risks associated with physical exertion, such as those listed in table 1.5, even though the effects tend to be as a result of an overexertion in either intensity, duration or both. It should be made clear that most of the evidence regarding physical activity and 'risk' relates to those injuries (regardless of the type) that occur as a result of playing sport (either competitive or recreational).

In sport, the competitive nature and forces involved mean that the risk of injury tends to be very high. In exercise-type activities such as gym and keep-fit, however, there tend to be fewer injuries, especially of the extrinsic kind (see table 1.5). It should also be pointed out that people who take part in moderate- to vigorous-intensity activities (either sport or exercise) have a higher risk of musculoskeletal injuries (injuries that affect bone or tissue such as muscle, tendon, ligament or cartilage) than those who take part in activity at lower intensities. Obviously the most serious injury as a result of physical exertion is death. Fortunately, sudden cardiac death, especially in younger people, is rare and in most cases (up to 500 every year in the UK) is thought to be caused by an underlying heart condition. Even though underlying heart problems may be the main cause of sudden cardiac death, fitness levels are also

Table 1.5	Potential risks associated with physical activity
Risk	**Explanation**
Musculoskeletal injuries	There are basically two forms of injury that can occur as a result of physical exertion. The first – 'extrinsic' injuries – are caused following some kind of external force such as a broken leg as a result of a tackle in football. The second – 'intrinsic' injuries – are caused by internal forces in the body such as too much strain being put on a muscle, which tears or ruptures.
Osteoarthritis	Injuries sustained during competitive sports have been shown to increase the risk of developing osteoarthritis. This can be due to repetitive movement resulting in wear or high impact resulting in direct damage.
Heart problems	Serious cardiac events such as heart attacks can occur with physical exertion. Unfortunately there have been many heart attack-related deaths over the years associated with both elite and non-elite sportspeople.
Addiction	People can become addicted to exercise and even experience withdrawal symptoms such as irritability and intolerance when they cannot exercise. Fortunately, the numbers of people who exercise to levels that cause health problems are, in percentage terms, very low.

thought to play an important role. For example, research by Albert and colleagues in 2000 showed that those who have low levels of regular vigorous activity are twice as likely to suffer sudden cardiac death during or after exercise compared to those who have high levels of regular vigorous physical activity. Interestingly, the research by Albert *et al.* also shows a gender difference, as men doing regular vigorous activities have the greatest risk compared to women, children and those doing regular moderate-intensity activities.

EXERCISE GUIDELINES

It is difficult to find exercise guidelines that are standardised across the globe, however the Department of Health's *Annual Report of the Chief Medical Officer* of 2009 compared general guidelines for moderate-intensity physical activity between the UK, USA and Australia. The guidelines, as can be seen in table 1.6, have been separated into those for children, younger adults and older adults.

The general physical activity guidelines for each special population chapter within this book (adapted from a variety of recognised sources) refer specifically to the intensity, duration and frequency of cardiovascular and resistance-type activities. It is useful, therefore, to have a better understanding of these terms as well as the term 'volume' of activity, which is used when talking about the risk of a condition.

Table 1.6	General guidelines for moderate-intensity physical activity		
	Children	**Young adults**	**Older adults**
England	60 minutes each day	30 minutes 5 times a week	30 minutes 5 times a week
Scotland	60 minutes on most days of the week	30 minutes on most days of the week	30 minutes on most days of the week + 3 bouts of strength and balance exercise a week
Wales	60 minutes 5 times a week	30 minutes 5 times a week	30 minutes 5 times a week
Northern Ireland	60 minutes each day	30 minutes 5 times a week	30 minutes 5 times a week
USA	60 minutes each day	150 minutes each week or 75 minutes of vigorous activity each week + strength activities 2 days a week	150 minutes each week or 75 minutes of vigorous activity each week + strength activities 2 days a week
Australia	60 minutes each day	30 minutes on most days of the week	30 minutes on most days of the week

INTENSITY

Most of the guidelines for physical activity (from internationally recognised sources) suggest moderate intensity levels, but this is often difficult to estimate as it can vary from one individual to another because intensity in most cases is usually based on heart rate. For example, a person who is unfit may only have to walk quickly to be at a moderate intensity level, whereas a very fit person may be able to run quite fast before they are at that same level. There are, however, many resources available that give examples of activities that are considered to be of light, moderate or vigorous intensity (and are usually based on a person of average weight and fitness). Table 1.7 is based on research by Ainsworth and colleagues in 2000; it shows common activities and the average intensity levels associated with them. The table also shows a measurement known as 'metabolic equivalents', or METs, which is a measure of how far energy expenditure (energy being used in the body) is raised above the resting level; 1 MET is the amount of energy being used by the body at rest (also known as the resting metabolic rate, or RMR). It follows therefore that 2 METs is simply double the amount of energy used at rest, and so on. As an example, the third column in table 1.7 shows the total energy expenditure for a person weighing 60 kg and exercising for 30 minutes (this is measured in kilocalories or kcals). As many food sources now have energy values in kcals (kilo simply means 1000) this helps people to estimate the energy value of their exercise for comparison purposes.

Table 1.7	Intensities and energy expenditure for common types of physical activity		
Common activity	**Intensity level**	**Intensity (METs)**	**Energy expenditure (kcal) 60 kg person 30 minutes' activity**
Ironing	Light	2.3	69
Cleaning	Light	2.5	75
Walking – 2 mph	Light	2.5	75
Painting/decorating	Moderate	3.0	90
Walking – 3 mph	Moderate	3.3	99
Vacuuming	Moderate	3.5	105
Golf walking, pulling clubs	Moderate	4.3	129
Badminton – social	Moderate	4.5	135
Tennis – doubles	Moderate	5.0	150
Walking – brisk, 4 mph	Moderate	5.0	150
Mowing lawn	Moderate	5.5	165
Cycling – 10–12 mph	Moderate	6.0	180
Aerobic dancing	Vigorous	6.5	195
Cycling – 12–14 mph	Vigorous	8.0	240
Swimming – slow crawl	Vigorous	8.0	240
Tennis – singles	Vigorous	8.0	240
Running – 6 mph	Vigorous	10.0	300
Running – 7 mph	Vigorous	11.5	345
Running – 8 mph	Vigorous	13.5	405

DURATION

Many recognised guidelines suggest that 30 minutes is the minimum amount of time a person should spend doing moderate-intensity activity, however this is not always possible due to the lifestyles of certain individuals. The reason for this is that it is thought that 30 minutes is the minimum amount of time that would result in any reasonable health-related benefits. There is a great deal of evidence to indicate that shorter bouts of activity accumulated throughout the day can be just as effective in terms of health-related benefits as a single longer bout. It should be emphasised, though, that 30 minutes is just a minimum guideline so it is important to remember that obese people may need up to 45–60 minutes or more of moderate-intensity physical activity a day to make substantial gains in weight loss. This is where several shorter bouts of activity accumulated throughout the day may make it easier for people to achieve these targets.

FREQUENCY

This is a relatively simple term that just means 'how often'. For example, the frequency could be on a daily basis, as in how many sessions per day, or it could be on a weekly basis, as in how many sessions per week. Both aerobic and resistance training sessions are usually prescribed in sessions per week.

VOLUME

In simple terms, the volume of activity refers to the duration and the intensity combined. Generally speaking, for certain conditions such as coronary heart disease and type 2 diabetes, the higher the volume of physical activity (or the higher the fitness level of the individual), the lower the risk of disease related to inactivity. This

effect can be seen in fig 1.2, and is also known as a 'dose-response' effect. In other words, the higher the dose (volume of physical activity, or fitness levels in this case) the greater the response (reduced risk of disease).

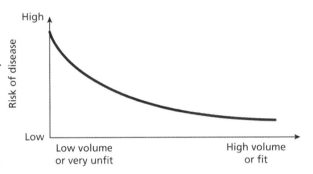

Figure 1.2 Risk of disease and the effect of physical activity or fitness level

RECOMMENDED READING

Ainsworth, B.E., Haskell, W.L., Whitt, M.C., Irwin, M.L., Swartz, A.M., Strath, S.J., O'Brien, W.L., Bassett, D.R., Schmitz, K.H., Emplaincourt, P.O., Jacobs, D.R. & Leon, A.S. (2000) Compendium of physical activities: an update of activity codes and MET intensities. *Medicine and Science in Sports and Exercise*, 32: S489–S504

Albert, C.M., Mittleman, M.A., Chae, C.U., Lee, I.M., Hennekens, C.H. & Manson, J.E. (2000) Triggering of sudden death from cardiac causes by vigorous exertion. *New England Journal of Medicine*, 343: 1355–1361

American College of Sports Medicine (2009a) *ACSM's exercise management for persons with chronic diseases and disabilities* (3rd edn). Champaign, IL: Human Kinetics

American College of Sports Medicine (2009a) *ACSM's guidelines for exercise testing and prescription* (8th edn). London: Lippincott Williams & Wilkins

Department for Culture, Media and Sport (2009) *Taking part: The national survey of culture, leisure and sport 2007–2008*. HMSO

Department of Health (2004) *At least 5 a week: Evidence on the impact of physical activity and its relationship to health*. London: Department of Health

Department of Health (2009) *Annual Report of the Chief Medical Officer*. London: Department of Health

Health Survey for England (2008) *Healthy lifestyles: Knowledge, attitudes and behaviour*. Leeds: NHS Information Centre for Health and Social Care

Health Survey for England (2006) *CVD and risk factors adults, obesity and risk factors children*. Leeds: NHS information Centre for Health and Social Care

NHS Information Centre, Lifestyle Statistics (2009) *Statistics on obesity, physical activity and diet: England, February 2009*. London: NHS Information Centre for Health and Social Care

World Health Organization (2002) *The World Health Report 2002. Reducing risks, promoting healthy life*. Geneva: WHO Press

USEFUL WEBSITES

Department for Culture, Media and Sport – www.culture.gov.uk

Department of Health – www.dh.gov.uk

NHS Information Centre – www.ic.nhs.uk

World Health Organization – www.who.int/en

OBESITY

2

KEYPOINTS

- In 2007, it was estimated that 24% of adults (aged 16 or over) in England were obese.
- Women were more likely than men to be morbidly obese (3% compared to 1%).
- 16.8% of boys aged 2–15 years and 16.1% of girls in the same age category were classed as obese.
- 37% of adults had a raised waist circumference in 2006 compared to 23% in 1993. Women were more likely than men to have a raised waist circumference (41% and 32% respectively).
- Of children aged 8 to 15 who were classed as obese, two-thirds (66%) of girls and 60% of boys thought that they were too heavy.
- Low levels of physical activity in England play a significant part in the increase of obesity.
- Physical activity can reduce risk of mortality and morbidity for those who are already overweight or obese.
- For people who are overweight or obese, a combination of physical activity and diet is recommended for weight loss.
- Achieving the recommendation of at least 30 minutes of at least moderate-intensity physical activity on five or more days a week is recommended as a minimum for weight loss, however 45–60 minutes of activity each day may be needed in order to prevent the development of obesity and those who have lost weight may need to do 60–90 minutes of activity a day in order to maintain their weight loss.
- Everyday activities such as brisk walking or cycling can be as effective for weight loss as supervised exercise programmes.

WHAT IS IT?

Generally speaking, the term obesity can be used to describe an individual who is carrying excess body weight in relation to their height. Wilmore and Costill (2007) are more specific in their definition, which states that an individual who has excessive amounts of body fat (more than 25% for

27

males and 35% for females) can be categorised as obese. In an attempt to take this a stage further, the American College of Sports Medicine (ACSM) has defined obesity as 'the percentage of body fat at which an individual's risk of disease increases'. One of the easiest methods (but not the most accurate) to indirectly measure body fat percentage is body mass index (BMI). BMI is a very common method, which simply divides a person's weight by their height squared (i.e. height multiplied by height).

Table 2.1	BMI classifications according to NICE guidelines (2010)
Classification	**BMI (kg/m²)**
Underweight	Less than 18.5
Healthy weight	18.5–24.9
Overweight	25–29.9
Obesity class I	30–34.9
Obesity class II	35–39.9
Obesity class III	40 or more

Body mass index formula

$$BMI = \frac{Weight\ (kg)}{Height\ squared\ (m^2)}$$

According to the National Institute for Health and Clinical Excellence (NICE), a BMI below 25 is considered to be low risk, whereas a BMI of 25 to 29.9 is classed as overweight, and 30 or above is classed as obese (see table 2.1). The problem with BMI is that it does not take into account body composition (fat and lean tissue), so an individual who has substantially increased their muscle mass through regular resistance training may have a BMI in the obese category but they would not be at the same risk as an individual with a similar BMI due to excess body fat. This method has also been shown to be inaccurate in women who are pregnant or breastfeeding, or those who are classed as being frail.

In terms of the causes of obesity, there are a number of specific genes associated with the condition, with suggestions that genetic factors may be linked to excess weight gain from the first few months of life. In fact, children of obese parents have a much higher risk of becoming obese than if their parents were of normal weight. In terms of food intake being the cause of obesity, it is only in relatively recent times (especially in developed countries) that energy-dense, low-cost food has been readily available, leading to overindulgence and hence weight gain. This is obviously proving easy to succumb to sensory factors such as sight, smell and taste, and the availability of food can increase appetite to such an extent that it becomes difficult to suppress; this common phenomenon is known as 'hedonic' hunger. There is a common misconception that obese people have slower metabolic rates (the amount of energy the body is using at any one time) than non-obese people. Unfortunately, many studies worldwide have suggested the opposite to be true in that energy usage at rest (known as resting metabolic rate) increases with body weight.

PREVALENCE

In 2009 the NHS Information Centre published a report which stated that, in 2007, 24% of adults in

England (that is 24% of men and 24% of women) were classified as obese. This is a 9% increase from the percentage of obese adults in England that was reported in 1993. The NHS report also stated that 16.8% of boys and 16.1% of girls aged 2–15 years were classed as obese, which had risen from 10.9% and 12.0% in 1995. The number of prescriptions for drugs to treat obesity was also reported to have risen, from 127,000 in 1999 to 1.23 million in 2007 (at a cost of £51.6 million). According to the House of Commons Health Committee in 2004, estimates of the cost of obesity in England in 2002 were £3.3–3.7 billion, including the direct costs of treating obesity and indirect costs including lost earnings from days off work. On a global scale, the World Health Organization reported that in 2010 China and Japan had obesity levels as low as 5% for adults, whereas Samoa had obesity levels of 75%. Perhaps the most frightening statistic is that, according to the NHS, one-third of children under the age of 11 years will be overweight by 2011 and, by 2025, it is estimated that 47% of males and 36% of females will be obese. As overweight and obesity are reaching epidemic levels, not only in the UK but on a global scale, it is worth summarising the findings of the 2009 NHS obesity report.

- In 2007, 24% of adults (aged 16 or over) in England were classified as obese (BMI of 30 kg/m^2 or over) – an overall increase from 15% in 1993.
- Men and women were equally likely to be obese, however men were more likely than women (41% compared to 32%) to be overweight (BMI of 25 to less than 30 kg/m^2).

- 37% of adults had a raised waist circumference in 2007 compared to 23% in 1993. Women were more likely than men (41% and 33% respectively) to have a raised waist circumference (over 88 cm in women, over 102 cm in men).
- Using both BMI and waist circumference to assess risk of health problems, for men: 19% were estimated to be at increased risk; 13% at high risk; and 21% at very high risk. Equivalent figures for women were: 15% at increased risk; 16% at high risk; and 23% at very high risk.
- In 2007, 17% of boys and 16% of girls aged 2 to 15 were classed as obese, an increase from 11% and 12% respectively in 1995. Indications suggest that the trend in obesity may be flattening out and the next couple of years' data will be important in confirming whether this is a continuing pattern.
- Boys were slightly more likely than girls to be overweight or obese (31% compared to 30%).
- In 2007, 1.23 million prescription items were dispensed for the treatment of obesity compared to 127,000 items in 1999. Between 2006 and 2007, the number of items dispensed for the treatment of obesity increased by 16% (from 1.06 million in 2006).

Finally, the 2009 NHS report shows how people in England are very much on a par with the rest of the world in terms of overweight and obesity in that 65% of men and 56% of women were overweight in 2007 (this is including those individuals who are obese). Unfortunately this means that less than half of the entire population in England are considered to be of a healthy weight, and this number is falling.

SYMPTOMS

Even though most people will associate overweight or obese people with being large, thinner people can also have a high percentage of body fat, so it is not always correct to assume that appearance can be a symptom resulting from overweight or obesity. As far as symptoms are concerned, there are no obvious ones that would relate to obesity alone. For example, most obese people would suffer breathlessness as a result of any physical activity or exertion, however this is usually as an indirect result of a low level of fitness rather than a direct result of being obese. As obesity is a major risk factor for many conditions, such as diabetes and hypertension, this will be discussed later in the relevant chapters rather than at this particular point.

DIAGNOSIS

When people are measured for overweight or obesity they are actually measured by whatever means in terms of body composition. The term body composition can be thought of (in simple terms, as it can be much more complicated) as the amount of fat tissue and the amount of lean tissue (everything that is not fat) within the body. Measurement of this is quite complicated as the only 'direct' way to measure true body composition is by dissection of cadavers (cutting up dead bodies) to see how much fat tissue there is. All other methods (see table 2.2 for a selection of the most common methods) of testing for body composition are based on estimates made from the few cadaver studies that have been carried out over the years, and are known as 'indirect' methods.

Table 2.2	Indirect methods of measuring body composition
Method	**Description**
Densitometry	For example, underwater weighing. The measurement of density is based on Archimedes' principle that 'a body immersed in a fluid is balanced by a buoyancy force equivalent to the weight of fluid displaced'. By measuring weight when submerged, a measure of an individual's body density can be found and converted to body fat percentage.
Plethysmography	This is measured by the amount of air displaced by the body, which is a similar principle to that of Archimedes. A person sits in a small chamber and the volume of air displaced is used to calculate body fat percentage.
Body imaging techniques	Dual-energy X-ray absorptiometry (DXA) and nuclear magnetic resonance (NMR) imaging are known as body imaging techniques. DXA works by analysing the passing of X-rays with low energy and high energy through the body. The passing of these X-rays depends on the composition of the tissues they pass through. NMR uses powerful magnetic fields, which provide a clearer picture of soft tissues than X-rays do.
Bioelectrical impedance	Bodystat® and other similar electrical devices in this category. It is based on the principle that an electric current flows more easily through water than fat so, depending on the current flow, body fat percentage can be calculated.
Anthropometry	Skinfold, height, body weight, girths, bone widths and BMI. For skinfold measurements, callipers (a device used to grip fat tissue) are used to measure the amount of fat at various sites on the body.

In terms of tests that can be done (for the purpose of measuring any improvement as a result of some sort of physical activity intervention), probably the most simple and least expensive to administer would be bioelectrical impedance and anthropometric measurements. If the tester takes baseline measurements (these are just measurements taken before any programme of activity has started) of an individual using whichever method they agree upon, follow-up testing could be done at regular intervals (such as 12-week periods). Repeating the tests at regular intervals can help the individual in many ways. For instance, based on the results of testing, goals could be set, which often helps to motivate the individual as they would have a specific target to follow and achieve. Follow-up testing can also help the activity supervisor as they should be able to gauge the success of the activity programme at regular intervals and change or adapt the programme if required. The testing procedures for bioelectrical impedance, skinfolds and waist-to-hip ratio (see below) are relatively straightforward to follow, so the reliability of the measurements should be consistent. The tester, however, needs to make sure that the equipment used in follow-up tests is the same as the equipment that was used for the first baseline test.

ELECTRICAL IMPEDANCE (BIOIMPEDANCE)

Bioelectrical impedance analysers are becoming a more frequently used method to assess body composition due to their ease of use, portability and relatively low cost. This type of measurement is based on the principle that the resistance to an electrical current is inversely related to the fat-free mass contained within the body. For example,

fat-free mass (such as muscle, bone and blood) contains virtually all of the water and electrolytes in the body and hence conducts most of the electric current produced by the bioelectrical analyser. Fat mass, on the other hand, is very low in water and electrolytes, and resists the flow of electric current. During testing, a small current (usually 0.4–0.8 amps) is passed between surface electrodes placed on the subject's hand and foot. The analyser then measures how much resistance (known as impedance) there is to this small current. The higher the resistance, the more fat tissue in the body there is, and the lower the resistance the more lean tissue there is. The analyser then calculates the information and displays this as a fat percentage. Commercially available analysers range from around £30 to several thousand pounds.

> The calculations done by the machine are gender and age specific and, as a consequence, some years ago it was found that going from the age of 29 to 30 saw a predicted body fat percentage increase by 4% overnight!

Care should be taken when using this method, however, as bioelectrical impedance values are largely determined by the amount of water in the body of the subject being tested and hence this must be standardised before any testing takes place. Testing should always be performed before any exercise and not when subjects are dehydrated because impedance can be greatly affected by fluid loss, changes in body temperature and sweat on the hands and legs. For this reason, make sure that when using this particular method, any pre-test instructions are repeated for follow-up tests.

Test box: Bioelectrical impedance

Equipment needed

There are several impedance analysers available on the market. The procedure for measurement is fairly simple but, regardless of the analyser used, the following preparation before testing, as recommended by Heyward in 1996, should be followed.

- No eating or drinking in the 4 hours before the test.
- No exercise for 12 hours before the test.
- Urinate within 30 minutes before the test.
- No alcohol consumption within 48 hours of the test.
- No diuretics (increases water loss) within 7 days before the test.

Test procedure

1. Subject should lie on a non-conductive surface (if you use a metal bench, ensure that it is covered with blankets and sheets).
2. Legs should be positioned such that the thighs do not touch, and hands positioned such that they do not touch the torso.
3. Position the electrodes with reference to the manufacturers' recommendations. This is usually relative to anatomical landmarks such as the ulnar head (wrist, as in fig 2.1a) and medial malleolus (ankle – as in fig 2.1b).
4. The electrode sites should be cleaned to reduce loss of signal and, depending on the type of electrode used, a conducting gel should be placed between the electrodes and the skin.
5. Follow the manufacturer's guidelines for measuring and record the result.

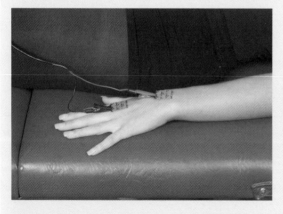 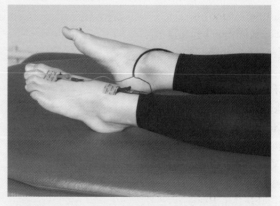

Figure 2.1a Electrode hand connections   **Figure 2.1b** Electrode foot connections

SKINFOLD TESTING

It is generally considered that, in the adult population, about 50–70% of adipose tissue is located subcutaneously (under the skin). This deposit of subcutaneous fat is assumed to be related to the deeper fat stores of the body and, because of this, skinfold measurement, using a device known as a skinfold calliper, has become a common and fairly reliable method of indirectly testing for body fat. A skinfold calliper is simply a device that is used to grip folds of fat tissue at various locations on the surface of the body. The precise location of the skinfold site (the point at which a skinfold measurement is taken) is vital as differences of as little as a centimetre can affect the values obtained for subjects, especially for sites around the abdominal area. There are several types of skinfold calliper that are commonly available. The choice of which to use is an important one, as calliper type can also affect the accuracy of the readings obtained. Harpenden, Lange and Holtain are three of the most recommended skinfold callipers, and cost between £100 and £200 to purchase. Cheaper plastic callipers such as the Slimguide are widely used even though they are less accurate and robust than the Harpenden callipers. They are, however, useful for training and are much cheaper at a cost of approximately £15. There are many methods of skinfold assessment that have been validated over the years. One of the most commonly used in health and fitness environments is the Durnin and Womersley four-site method developed in 1974, which is explained in the test box on page 34 and in table 2.3. Because of the potential for error that can occur when carrying out skinfold measurements (especially between different testers), it is important that pre-test conditions are adhered to in order to help reduce the potential measurement errors, and increase the reliability and reproducibility of future measurements.

Pre-test conditions

- Ensure that a warm, well-lit room is used and privacy is assured at all times for the subject being tested.
- If the assessor is male, measurements of females and children should be made sensitively, and supervised if possible.
- The subject should be as relaxed and as comfortable as possible (swimsuits – two-piece in the case of women – are ideal, although a vest and shorts may also be suitable for females).
- Subjects should always be clearly informed about the procedures involved in the testing and should be provided with an informed consent form to complete before participation in the test.
- All measurements should be made on the right-hand side of the body for standardisation purposes.

To find the body fat percentage, once all of the skinfold measurements have been taken, the individual measurement from all four sites should then be added together to give a total figure in millimetres. Then using table 2.4, find the total millimetre figure in the SUM column and read across to the appropriate age column (for men or women, depending on the subject) to give the body fat percentage. Note that the SUM column goes up in multiples, so a 'guesstimation' of the actual body fat percentage might be needed.

Test box: Skinfolds (Durnin and Womersley, 1974)

Equipment needed

Skinfold callipers, tape measure, marker pen.

Testing procedure

- The tester should raise a skinfold between the thumb and forefinger at the marked site following the natural cleavage lines of the skin (fig 2.2a).
- Use a rolling and pulling action to separate the fold from the muscle beneath.
- The calliper blades are applied perpendicularly to the fold and 1 cm away from the thumb and forefinger (fig 2.2b).
- Pressure is released. Record value 2 seconds later to the nearest 0.2 mm.
- All skin-folds should be measured three times with a 2-minute recovery to allow compression of the tissue to return to normal. Measure three times and use the median (middle) value obtained.
- Measure the four sites shown in table 2.3: biceps, triceps, subscapula, suprailiac.

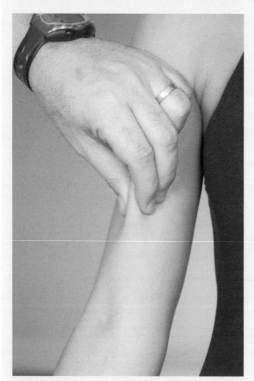

Figure 2.2a Grasping a skin fold

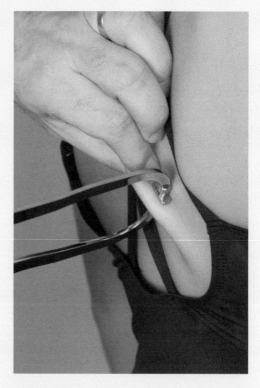

Figure 2.2b Calliper placement

Table 2.3	**Durnin and Womersley skinfold site locations**	
Subscapular	Oblique fold 2 cm below and 2 cm lateral to the inferior angle of the scapula at about 45° to the horizontal plane following the natural cleavage lines of the skin.	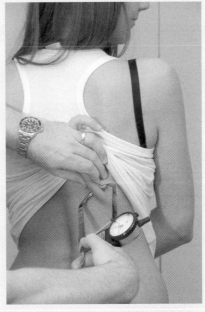
Triceps	Vertical fold raised on the posterior aspect of the triceps, exactly halfway between the olecranon process and the acromion process. Palms face forward.	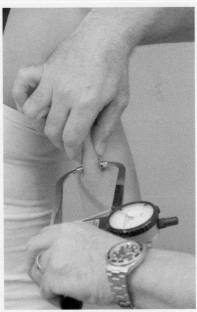

Table 2.3	Durnin and Womersley skinfold site locations (continued)
Biceps	Vertical fold on the anterior aspect of the biceps, at the same horizontal level as the triceps skinfold.
Suprailiac	Diagonal fold above the crest of the ilium at the point where an imaginary line would come down from the anterior axillary border. Slightly anterior to the iliac crest.

Table 2.4 Skinfold conversion table

MEN				WOMEN			
SUM				SUM			
(mm)	16–29	30–49	50+	(mm)	16–29	30–49	50+
20	8.1	12.1	12.5	14	9.4	14.1	17.0
22	9.2	13.2	13.9	16	11.2	15.7	18.6
24	10.2	14.2	15.1	18	12.7	17.1	20.1
26	11.2	15.2	16.3	20	14.1	18.4	21.4
28	12.1	16.1	17.4	22	15.4	19.5	22.6
30	12.9	16.9	18.5	24	16.5	20.6	23.7
35	14.7	18.7	20.8	26	17.6	21.5	24.8
40	16.3	20.3	22.8	28	18.6	22.4	25.7
45	17.7	21.8	24.7	30	19.5	23.3	26.6
50	19.0	23.0	26.3	35	21.6	25.2	28.6
55	20.2	24.2	27.8	40	23.4	26.8	30.3
60	21.2	25.3	29.1	45	25.0	28.3	31.9
65	22.2	26.3	30.4	50	26.5	29.6	33.2
70	23.2	27.2	31.5	55	27.8	30.8	34.6
75	24.0	28.0	32.6	60	29.1	31.9	35.7
80	24.8	28.8	33.7	65	30.2	32.9	36.7
85	25.6	29.6	34.6	70	31.2	33.9	37.7
90	26.3	30.3	35.5	75	32.2	34.7	38.6
95	27.0	31.0	36.5	80	33.1	35.6	39.5
100	27.6	31.7	37.3	85	34.0	36.3	40.4
110	28.8	32.9	38.8	90	34.8	37.1	41.1
120	29.9	34.0	40.2	95	35.6	37.8	41.9
130	31.0	35.0	41.5	100	36.3	38.5	42.6
140	31.9	36.0	42.8	110	37.7	39.7	43.9
150	32.8	36.8	43.9	120	39.0	40.8	45.1
160	33.6	37.7	45.0	130	40.2	41.9	46.2
170	34.4	38.5	46.0	140	41.3	42.9	47.3
180	35.2	39.2	47.0	150	42.3	43.8	48.2
190	35.9	39.9	47.9	160	43.2	44.7	49.1
200	36.5	40.6	48.8	170	44.6	45.5	50.0

WAIST-TO-HIP RATIO (WHR)

Not only is the quantity of fat an individual has linked with disease, but the location of that fat is also linked to disease. In fact, central fat mass is recognised as an independent risk factor for cardiovascular disease. However, WHR is partly dependent on the structure of the pelvis and muscle distribution, and has thus been questioned by some as a reliable measure of body composition. Waist circumference is commonly known as a more superior predictor of abdominal body fat and risk factor for CHD, so the tester could simply take the waist measurement and set targets to improve this. One of the advantages of using waist circumference over WHR is that only one measurement is taken and hence this reduces the risk of measurement error. Even though WHR is no longer recommended by the American Heart Association, in contrast to this some researchers in London have found WHR to be a good predictor of mortality in those individuals over the age of 75 years. However, if the tester decides to use WHR then the process in the test box below should be followed.

Test box: Waist-to-hip ratio

Resources required
Tape measure.

Test procedure
- Stand erect, abdomen and buttocks relaxed, arms at side and feet together.
- Measure the waist at its narrowest point and the hips at the widest point.
- Waist circumference is measured midway between the lower rib margin and the iliac crest in the horizontal plane (fig 2.3a).
- While the subject is standing, hip circumference is measured at the point yielding the maximum circumference over the buttocks using a tape measure to measure to the nearest 0.1 cm (fig 2.3b).
- Divide the waist measurement by the hip measurement.

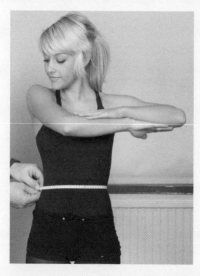

Figure 2.3a Waist measurement

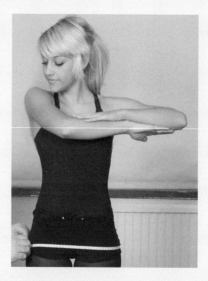

Figure 2.3b Hip measurement

Classification

According to the World Health Organization (WHO), a waist circumference of greater than 102 cm (40 inches) for males and 88 cm (35 inches) for females is an indication of an increased risk of developing type 2 diabetes, coronary heart disease and/or hypertension. There are also other sources of age-related risk categories, such as those listed in table 2.5, that have similar values across the ranges.

Table 2.5	Risk categories for waist-to-hip ratio scores				
Gender	Age	Low risk	Moderate risk	High risk	Very high risk
Men	20–29	<0.83	0.83–0.88	0.89–0.94	>0.94
	30–39	<0.84	0.84–0.91	0.92–0.96	>0.96
	40–49	<0.88	0.88–0.95	0.96–1.00	>1.00
	50–59	<0.90	0.90–0.96	0.97–1.02	>1.02
	60–69	<0.91	0.91–0.98	0.99–1.03	>1.03
Women	20–29	<0.71	0.71–0.77	0.78–0.82	>0.82
	30–39	<0.72	0.72–0.78	0.79–0.84	>0.84
	40–49	<0.73	0.73–0.79	0.80–0.87	>0.87
	50–59	<0.74	0.74–0.81	0.82–0.88	>0.88
	60–69	<0.76	0.76–0.83	0.84–0.90	>0.90

There are also risk tables available for measurements of waist circumference alone, such as those published by the American College of Sports Medicine (ACSM) in 2009. This can provide a very simple option for the tester, as waist measurement alone is considered to be a reasonable indication of the risk of certain diseases, such as type 2 diabetes and CHD. Taking only one measurement can also be easier for the subject to remember and focus on as opposed to having to remember two different measurements. Table 2.6 shows the waist circumference risk table adapted from the ACSM.

Table 2.6	Risk categories for waist circumference scores			
	Men		Women	
Risk	cm	inches	cm	inches
Very high	>120	>47	>110	>43.5
High	100–120	39.5–47	90–110	35.5–43.5
Low	80–99	31.5–39	70–89	28.5–35
Very low	<80	<31.5	<70	<28.5

Table 2.7	NICE risk categories for BMI and waist circumference		
	Waist circumference		
	Low	*High*	*Very high*
Male	<94 cm	94–102 cm	>102 cm
Female	<80 cm	80–88 cm	>88 cm
Normal weight	No increased risk	No increased risk	Increased risk
Overweight (BMI of 25 to less than 30)	No increased risk	Increased risk	High risk
Obesity I (BMI of 30 to less than 35)	Increased risk	High risk	Very high risk

Some other guidelines go even further than using just one method to assess the risk of health problems associated with obesity. For example, the NICE guidelines on prevention, identification, assessment and management of overweight and obesity suggest that the risk of the associated health problems should be identified using a combination of BMI and waist circumference for those people with a BMI of less than 35 kg/m². This is because, for adults with a BMI of 35 kg/m² or more, it is assumed that the risks are very high regardless of waist circumference measurement. Table 2.7 shows the category of risk calculated from the combination of BMI and waist circumference measurements.

RISK FACTORS

Although the causes of overweight and obesity can include hypothalamic, endocrine and genetic disorders, diet and physical inactivity are generally considered to be the prime causes or risk factors for overweight and obesity. It is important therefore that physical activity is promoted as an essential requirement for everyone as it has been shown that regular physical activity reduces the risk of individuals becoming obese by 50% compared to those individuals who have sedentary lifestyles. Overweight and obesity are often linked to many other health problems that are related to the excess body fat of the individual. According to McArdle, Katch and Katch (2006), there are ten main health consequences that are likely to occur at some stage in obese individuals. These are:

1 Cardiovascular disease (CVD)
2 Type 2 diabetes
3 Hypertension (high blood pressure)
4 Dyslipidaemia (high blood lipids)
5 Stroke
6 Apnoea during sleep (breathing stops for a few seconds)
7 Degenerative joint problems
8 Some types of cancer
9 Gallstones
10 Infertility

The seriousness of the related health problems is evident as, according to the Department of Health in 2004, obesity was responsible for over 9000 premature deaths in England every year (the link between BMI and mortality can be seen in fig 2.4). Obesity has also been suggested by many research studies to be one of the primary causes of type 2 diabetes, yet a reduction of only 5% of body weight (which is very achievable for most obese people) can prevent most of those who are obese and have impaired glucose tolerance from developing type 2 diabetes. Furthermore, it has been shown that a reduction of body weight in overweight and obese individuals with type 2 diabetes is associated with a reduction in mortality. There is also a strong relationship between obesity and CVD, and the level of obesity can be used to predict CVD, particularly for women. In other words, the larger the percentage of body fat the higher the risk of developing CVD. A similar relationship has also been found between obesity and death rates from all cancers.

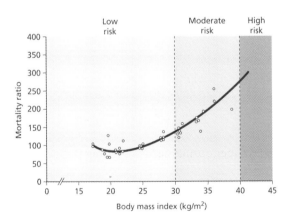

Figure 2.4 BMI and the risk of mortality

PHYSICAL ACTIVITY BENEFITS

It is generally accepted and recommended by the ACSM that a combination of an increase in calorie expenditure (physical activity) and a decrease in calorie intake (eating food) is the most effective method for the treatment of overweight and obesity in the long term. In scientific terms this relates to the first law of thermodynamics, which basically states that 'energy can neither be created nor destroyed'. In terms of overweight or obesity, this means that any food taken into the body is a source of energy that can either be stored or used as a fuel supply for physical activity purposes. If the energy is stored, it can easily be stored as fat. If the energy is used for physical activity, however, it is first converted to chemical energy to help the muscles do the activity and then most is lost as heat (as we are not very efficient beings). In simple terms, to lose weight, energy expenditure must be greater than energy input. Many guidelines therefore recommend a combination of diet and physical activity for weight loss, although there are other benefits associated with this weight loss, such as:

- reduction in the loss of fat tissue,
- maintenance of resting metabolic rate (RMR),
- improvement in blood lipids,
- maintenance of long-term weight loss,
- improved self-esteem and
- improved self-image.

As a long-term health benefit, it has been suggested that about 35% of all deaths caused by CHD and diabetes mellitus, and about 32% of all deaths caused by colon cancer, could be avoided if everyone took part in some form of regular physical activity that would be classified as vigorous (a good reason to promote all forms of exercise). It will come as no surprise therefore to know that inactive people are more likely to be overweight or obese than are active people. Many research studies, such as those by Schultz and Schoeller (1994) and Westerterp and Goran (1997), show that there is an association between energy expenditure and lower fat mass. In other words, those with higher levels of energy expenditure tend to have a lower body-fat percentage. There are also studies that have shown a link between fitness levels and substantial weight gain. For example, studies by Fogelholm and Kukkonen-Harjula (2000) and Di Pietro (1999) have shown that higher fitness levels can help to reduce weight gain. There is also a suggestion that more time spent inactive leads to a greater body-fat percentage, as demonstrated in studies such as those by Martínez-González et al. (1999) and Brown et al. (2003). It is commonly agreed that by physical activity alone it is difficult to achieve weight loss, therefore a combination of a healthy diet and an increased level of physical activity is always advised. For example, many studies, such as those by Blair and Bouchard (1999), Ross et al. (2000, 2004), Ross and Janssen (2001), and Mulvihil and Quigley (2003), show that physical activity alone results in only modest weight loss of around 0.5–1 kg per month, whereas a combination of increased physical activity and reduced calorie intake results in a much greater weight loss. Even though studies have taken place over various lengths of time with varying results, in general it is agreed that the greater the level of physical activity (higher energy expenditure), the greater the overall weight loss – especially if combined with a healthy eating regime.

PHYSICAL ACTIVITY GUIDELINES

Many of the guidelines relating to physical activity for weight loss agree that aerobic-type activity combined with light resistance training is optimal for this particular population as the main goal is one of increased energy expenditure. Walking is often the best way in which to begin a physical activity programme as most individuals in this population are not embarrassed by it and therefore have more chance of participating in the longer term. Supervisors should also encourage more expenditure in daily routines such as parking at the furthest end of car parks, using stairs rather than lifts and getting up to change the TV channel. It should be noted, though, that there is a high drop-out rate with this population, therefore short-term goals should be used and supervisors should be constantly trying to find ways to motivate the individual. It is recommended that people in this particular population seek clearance from their GP before undertaking any programme of physical activity, to make sure that there are no other underlying problems that may be made worse by the activities. Table 2.8 gives the general physical activity guidelines for those who are obese.

The majority of health or fitness instructors (and even those supervising) will at some stage work with obese (or at least overweight) individuals. Even though individuals in this population will have their own specific goals and progress at different rates in relation to intensity and duration etc., table 2.9 shows how a general cardiovascular training programme can be progressed for the majority of individuals in this population who have no recent history of physical activity.

Table 2.8	Physical activity guidelines for obesity	
	Aerobic training	**Strength training**
Mode	• Because of the stress on the joints, low-impact activities should be chosen (walking, swimming)	• In the initial stages, this may involve callisthenics to provide overload, but the client may then move on to resistance equipment
Intensity	• Low to moderate intensity • 40–85%HRmax • 6–15 RPE	• Use loads within the individual's capability • Overload by increasing intensity gradually
Duration	• 20–60 minutes per session • Increase intensity with slow progression	• Perform 1 to 3 sets of 12–15 RM • 1–2 minutes' rest between exercises
Frequency	• At least 5 days per week	• 2–3 sessions per week
Precautions	• Avoid impact activities • Use non-weight-bearing alternatives • The expenditure should be approximately 150–400 kcals per day	• Avoid impact or jarring exercises

General precautions

• It is recommended that a dual approach be adopted: increase caloric expenditure and decrease caloric intake (no less than 1200 kcal/day)
• Negative energy balance (calories in minus calories out) of 500–1000 kcal/day
• Aim for a maximum weight loss of 1 kg/week
• Obese people have an increased risk of hyperthermia, so watch out for overheating

Table 2.9	Training progressions for sedentary low-risk participants			
Programme stage	**Week**	**Sessions per week**	**Activity intensity (%HRmax)**	**Activity duration (mins)**
Initial stage	1	3	40–50	15–20
	2	3–4	40–50	20–25
	3	3–4	50–60	20–25
	4	3–4	50–60	25–30
Improvement stage	5–7	3–4	60–70	25–30
	8–10	3–4	60–70	30–35
	11–13	3–4	65–75	30–35
	14–16	3–5	65–75	30–35
	17–20	3–5	70–85	35–40
	21–24	3–5	70–85	35–40
Maintenance stage	24+	3–5	70–85	20–60

This is a general programme which assumes that, during the initial stage (first four weeks) of a physical activity programme, individuals will be unfit. For this reason, the intensity level should be kept quite low and the duration short. Any progression should be done in small amounts and the individual should be asked constantly if they are able to cope. As with any individual, a maximum goal should be agreed and, when reached, a maintenance level of activity should then be undertaken in order to help create a regular lifestyle routine.

RECOMMENDED READING

American College of Sports Medicine. (2001) Appropriate intervention strategies for weight loss and prevention of weight regain for adults. Position Stand. *Medicine and Science in Sports and Exercise*, 33: 2145–2156

American College of Sports Medicine (2009a) *ACSM's exercise management for persons with chronic diseases and disabilities* (3rd edn). Champaign, IL: Human Kinetics

American College of Sports Medicine (2009b) *ACSM's guidelines for exercise testing and prescription* (8th edn). London: Lippincott Williams & Wilkins

Astrup, A. & Finer, N. (2000) Redefining type 2 diabetes: 'Diabesity' or 'obesity dependent diabetes mellitus'? *Obesity Reviews*, 1: 57–59

Blair, S.N. & Bouchard, C. (1999) Physical activity in the prevention and treatment of obesity and its comorbidities: American College of Sports Medicine Consensus Conference (Roundtable Preface). *Medicine and Science in Sports and Exercise*, 31: S497

Bouchard, C., Shephard, R.J. & Stephens, T. (1994) *Physical activity, fitness and health. International proceedings and consensus statement.* Champaign, IL: Human Kinetics

Bouchard, C. & Tremblay, A. (1997) Genetic influences on the response of body fat and fat distribution to positive and negative energy balances in human identical twins. *Journal of Nutrition*, 127: 943S–947S

British Heart Foundation Health Promotion Research Group (2005) *Coronary heart disease statistics*. University of Oxford: Department of Public Health

Brown, W.J., Miller, Y.D. & Miller, R. (2003) Sitting time and work patterns as indicators of overweight and obesity in Australian youth. *International Journal of Obesity*, 27: 1340–1346

Butland, B., Kopelman, P., McPherson, K., Thomas, S., Mardell, J. & Parry, V. (2007) *Foresight. Tackling obesities: future choices – project report* (2nd edn). London: Government Office for Science

Camilo, D., Ribeiro, J., Toro, A., Baracat, E. & Filho, A. (2010) Obesity and asthma: Association or coincidence? *Journal of Paediatrics*, 86(1): 6–14

Deckelbaum, R. & Williams, C. (2001) Childhood obesity: The health issue. *Obesity Research*, 9(4): 239–243

Dehghan, M., Danesh, N. & Merchant, A.T. (2005) Childhood obesity, prevalence and prevention. *Nutrition Journal*, 4: 24

Dehghan, M. & Merchant, A.T. (2008) Is bioelectrical impedance accurate for use in large epidemiological studies? *Nutrition Journal*, 7: 26

De Lorenzo, A., Bertini, I., Candeloro, N., Iacopino, L., Andreoli, A. & Van Loan, M. (1998) Comparison of different techniques to measure body composition in moderately active adolescents. *British Journal of Sports Medicine*, 32: 215–219

Department of Health (2004) *Choosing health: Making healthy choices easier*. London: HMSO

Department of Health (2006) *Health Survey for England 2006: CVD and risk factors adults, obesity and risk factors children*. London: HMSO

Di Pietro, L. (1999) Physical activity in the prevention of obesity: Current evidence and research issues. *Medicine and Science in Sports and Exercise*, 31: S542–S546

Di Pietro, L., Kohl, H.W., Barlow, C.E. & Blair, S.N. (1998) Improvements in cardiorespiratory fitness attenuate age-related weight gain in healthy men and women: The Aerobics Centre Longitudinal Study. *International Journal of Obesity*, 22: 55–62

Donnelly, J.E., Jacobsen, D.J., Heelan, K.S., Seip, R. & Smith, S. (2000) The effects of 18 months of intermittent vs continuous exercise on aerobic capacity, body weight and composition, and metabolic fitness in previously sedentary, moderately obese females.

International Journal of Obesity and Related Metabolic Disorders, 24: 566–572

Drøyvold, W.B., Holmen, J., Midthjell, K. & Lydersen, S. (2004) BMI change and leisure time physical activity (LTPA): An 11-y follow-up study in apparently healthy men aged 20–69y with normal weight at baseline. *International Journal of Obesity*, 28: 410–417

Durnin, J.V.G.A. & Womersley, J. (1974) Body fat assessed from total body density and its estimation from skinfold thickness: Measurements on 481 men and women aged from 16 to 72 years. *British Journal of Nutrition*, 32: 77

Farooqi, S. & O'Rahilly, S. (2006) Genetics of obesity in humans. *Endocrine Reviews*, 27(7): 710–718

Fogelholm, M. & Kukkonen-Harjula, K. (2000) Does physical activity prevent weight gain: A systematic review. *Obesity Reviews*, 1: 95–111

Gaziano, J.M. (2010) Fifth phase of the epidemiologic transition: The age of obesity and inactivity. *Journal of the American Medical Association*, 303(3): 275–276

Hager, R.L. (2006) Television viewing and physical activity in children. *Journal of Adolescent Health*, 39(5): 656–661

Health Survey for England (2007) *Healthy lifestyles: Knowledge, attitudes and behaviour.* Leeds: NHS Information Centre for Health and Social Care

Heyward, V.H. (1996) *Advance Fitness Assessment and Exercise Prescription.* Champaign: Human Kinetics

Hillsdon, M., Foster, C. & Thorogood, M. (2005, 2006) Interventions for promoting physical activity (Review). *Cochrane Database of Systematic Reviews*, 1: CD 003180

Hubert, H.B., Feinleib, M., McNemara, P.M. & Castelli, W.P. (1983) Obesity as an independent risk factor for cardiovascular disease: A 26-year follow-up of participants in the Framingham Heart Study. *Circulation*, 67: 968–977

Kamimura, M., Avesani, C., Cendoroglo, M., Canziani, M., Draibe, A. & Cuppari, L. (2003) Comparison of skinfold thicknesses and bioelectrical impedance analysis with dual-energy X-ray absorptiometry for the assessment of body fat in patients on long term haemodialysis therapy. *Nephrology Dialysis Transplantation*, 18: 101–105

Kotani, K., Nishida, M. & Yamashita, S. (1997) Two decades of annual medical examinations in Japanese obese children: Do obese children grow into obese adults? *International Journal of Obesity Related Metabolic Disorders*, 21: 912–921

Lobstein, T. & Frelut, M.L. (2003) Prevalence of overweight among children in Europe. *Obesity Reviews*, 4(4): 195–200

Martínez-González, M.Á., Martínez, J.A., Hu, F.B., Gibney, M.J. & Kearney, J. (1999) Physical inactivity, sedentary lifestyle and obesity in the European Union. *International Journal of Obesity*, 23: 1192–1201

McArdle, W.D., Katch, F.I. & Katch, V.L. (2006) *Essentials of exercise physiology* (3rd edn). Baltimore, MD: Lippincott Williams & Wilkins

McInnis, K.J. (2000) Exercise and obesity. *Coronary Artery Disease*, 11(2): 111–116

Mulvihill, C. & Quigley, R. (2003) The management of obesity and overweight: An analysis of reviews of diet, physical activity and behavioural approaches. *Evidence briefing* (1st edn). London: Health Development Agency

National Institute for Health and Clinical Excellence (2008) *Promoting and creating built or natural environments that encourage and support physical activity* (NICE public health guidance 8). London: NICE

NHS Information Centre, Lifestyle Statistics (2009) *Statistics on obesity, physical activity and diet: England, February 2009.* London: NHS Information Centre for Health and Social Care

Peterson, L., Schnor, P. & Sorenson, T.I.A. (2004) Longitudinal study of the long-term relationship between physical activity and obesity in adults. *International Journal of Obesity*, 28: 105–112

Pinkney, J., Wilding, J., Williams, G. & MacFarlane, I. (2002) Hypothalamic obesity in humans: What do we know and what can be done? *Obesity Reviews*, 3: 27–34

Prentice, A.M. & Jebb, S.A. (2001) Beyond body mass index. *Obesity Reviews*, 2(3): 141–147

Puhl, R.M. & Heuer, C.A. (2009) The stigma of obesity: A review and update. *Obesity Reviews*, 17: 941–964

Reilly, J.J., Methven, E., McDowell, Z.C., Alexander, D.A., Hacking, B., Stewart, L. & Kelnar, C. (2003) Health consequences of obesity: Systematic review. *Archives of Disease in Childhood*, 88: 748–752

Ricciardi, R. & Talbot, L. (2007) Use of bioelectrical impedance analysis in the evaluation, treatment, and prevention of overweight and obesity. *Journal of the American Academy of Nurse Practitioners*, 19(5): 235–241

Ross, R. & Janssen, I. (2001) Physical activity, total and regional obesity: Dose response considerations. *Medicine and Science in Sports and Exercise*, 33: S521–S527

Ross, R., Dagnone, D., Jones, P.J.H., Smith, H., Paddags, A., Hudson, R. & Janssen, I. (2000) Reduction in obesity and related comorbid conditions after diet-induced weight loss or exercise-induced weight loss in men. *Annals of Internal Medicine*, 133(2): 92–103

Ross, R., Janssen, I., Dawson, J., Kungl, A.M., Kuk, J.L., Wong, S.L., Nguyen-Duy, T.B., Lee, S., Kilpatrick, K. & Hudson, R. (2004) Exercise-induced reduction in obesity and insulin resistance in women: A randomized controlled trial. *Obesity Research*, 12(5): 789–798

Schulz, L.O. & Schoeller, D.A. (1994) A compilation of total daily energy expenditures and body weights in healthy adults. *American Journal of Clinical Nutrition*, 60: 676–681

Slentz, C.A., Duscha, B.D., Johnson, J.L., Ketchum, K., Aiken, L.B., Samsa, G.P., Houmard, J.A., Bales, C.W. & Kraus, W.E. (2004) Effects of the amount of exercise on body weight, body composition, and measures of central obesity. *Archives of Internal Medicine*, 164(1): 31–39

Story, M., Sallis, J. & Orleans, T. (2009) Adolescent obesity: Towards evidence based policy and environmental solutions. *Journal of Adolescent Health*, 45: S1–S5

Westerterp, K.R. & Goran, M.I. (1997) Relationship between physical activity related energy expenditure and body composition: A gender difference. *International Journal of Obesity*, 21: 184–188

Williamson, D.F., Thompson, T.J., Thun, M., Flanders, D., Pamuk, E. & Byers, T. (2000) Intentional weight loss and mortality among overweight individuals with diabetes. *Diabetes Care*, 23(10): 1499–1504

Wilmore, J.H. & Costill, D.L. (2007) *Physiology of sport and exercise* (4th edn). Champaign, IL: Human Kinetics

World Cancer Research Fund/American Institute for Cancer Research (2007) *Food, nutrition, physical activity, and the prevention of cancer: A global perspective.* Washington, DC: AICR

Woolf-May, K. (2006) *Exercise prescription: Physiological foundations.* London: Churchill Livingstone, Elsevier

World Health Organization (2005) *The challenge of obesity in the WHO European Region and the strategies for response.* Denmark: WHO Press

World Health Organization (2007) *The world health report 2007 – a safer future: Global public health security in the 21st century.* Geneva: WHO Press

USEFUL WEBSITES

American College of Sports Medicine – www.acsm.org

British Heart Foundation – www.bhf.org.uk

Department of Health – www.dh.gov.uk

National Institute for Health and Clinical Excellence – www.nice.org.uk

National Obesity Forum – www.nationalobesityforum.org.uk

NHS Information Centre – www.ic.nhs.uk

World Health Organization – www.who.int/en

DIABETES MELLITUS

3

KEYPOINTS

- In the UK around 1.4–1.6 million people have been diagnosed with diabetes.
- Type 2 diabetes often has few symptoms in the early stages, and it is estimated that half of those with type 2 diabetes have not yet been diagnosed.
- The last 30 years has seen a threefold increase in the number of cases of childhood diabetes.
- Obesity levels have also risen dramatically, which has impacted on numbers of type 2 diabetics, as it is estimated that about 80% of type 2 diabetics are obese.
- Worldwide, it is estimated that in 2010 there were approximately 285 million people with type 2 diabetes. This figure is expected to increase to 438 million people by 2030.
- About 5% of people in England have diabetes, which is more than in Scotland, Wales and Northern Ireland.
- Physical inactivity is a major risk factor for the development of type 2 diabetes.
- Physically active people have a 33–50% lower risk of developing type 2 diabetes compared with inactive people. The preventive effect is particularly strong for those at high risk of developing type 2 diabetes as it can reduce their risk of developing the disease by up to 64%.
- Among people with type 2 diabetes, regular moderate-intensity physical activity carried out three times a week can produce small but significant improvements in blood glucose control. Both aerobic and resistance exercise programmes produce similar benefits. Higher levels of intensity of physical activity produce greater benefits.
- Moderate to high levels of physical fitness appear to reduce the risk of all-cause mortality in patients with type 2 diabetes.

WHAT IS IT?

The correct term for this particular condition is 'diabetes mellitus', but for the purposes of this book it will be referred to just as 'diabetes'. Diabetes mellitus (which translates roughly from Greek and Latin as 'honey urine') is what is known as a metabolic disease and is concerned with the regulation, and in particular the storage, of blood sugar in the body. Blood sugar (known as 'glucose') is broken down from the carbohydrates we eat. When we eat carbohydrates in fruit, vegetables, pasta, bread etc., they are digested in the body to become glucose, which is absorbed into the bloodstream. This is why it is referred to as blood glucose, which is the main fuel for the brain and also for working muscles in the body, and is normally kept at a constant level either at rest or during any physical exertion. In order to keep blood glucose at the required level, various hormones (these are just chemical messengers) are released that control this process. The two main hormones that help regulate blood glucose are insulin and glucagon. Insulin is a hormone produced by specialised cells (called beta cells) in an organ in the body called the pancreas, located just behind the stomach, as can be seen in fig 3.1.

When the blood glucose level rises too high (hyperglycaemia, as this condition is known), normally as a result of an intake of food, the pancreas reacts to this by secreting the hormone insulin into the bloodstream. The insulin has the effect of lowering the blood glucose level to maintain it within the limits preferred by the body by transporting the glucose out of the blood and into organs and muscle cells. The hormone glucagon has the opposite effect when blood glucose levels are low. Diabetes is a condition in which the pancreas has a deficiency in insulin production or where there is no effect as a result of the insulin secreted. If an individual has any of these conditions they will be unable to regulate blood sugar levels, leading to either high blood glucose levels (hyperglycaemia) or low blood glucose levels (hypoglycaemia). There are, however, a variety of other terms that are used in

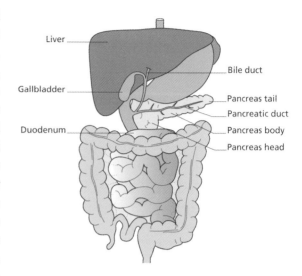

Figure 3.1 Location of the pancreas

relation to this disease. 'Insulin sensitivity', or 'insulin resistance', refers to how sensitive the organs and muscle cells are to the action of insulin. 'Glucose tolerance', on the other hand, refers to how well the body can ingest and store the glucose. Long-term effects of this condition can lead to other conditions, such as:

- blindness
- kidney failure
- nerve dysfunction
- heart problems
- blood vessel deterioration.

Depending on the behaviour of the condition there are essentially two main categories of diabetes, known as type 1 diabetes and type 2 diabetes, and a less common category known as gestational diabetes. There is also a condition known as 'impaired glucose tolerance', which refers to people who do not have normal glucose regulation but have not quite reached the stage of diabetes. Impaired glucose tolerance usually precedes type 2 diabetes.

TYPE 1: INSULIN DEPENDENT DIABETES MELLITUS (IDDM)

This type of diabetes is also known as juvenile-onset diabetes as it occurs primarily in the younger age population. Individuals with this particular type of diabetes are dependent on regular injections of insulin as their own pancreas cannot secrete any. The condition known as 'ketoacidosis' is reported to be very common with this type of diabetes; this is where the lack of glucose transport to the muscle cells leads to development of ketone bodies, which have a toxic effect and can be lifethreatening as they can lower the pH (acidity level) of the blood. Figures usually show that about 5–10% of diabetics are type 1.

TYPE 2: NON-INSULIN DEPENDENT DIABETES MELLITUS (NIDDM)

This type of diabetes is also known as adult- or maturity-onset diabetes as it occurs primarily in the older age population, even though the number of children who are developing type 2 diabetes is rising. Those with type 2 diabetes do not require any insulin injections to manage their glucose levels. This particular type of diabetes is related to the lack of ability of the organs and muscles of the body to take in and store glucose. In other words, the condition is mainly due to a resistance to insulin. Type 2 diabetes is also very closely linked with obesity, therefore the primary treatment that is generally recommended is a combination of dietand physical activity to help regulate blood glucose levels and reduce body fat. Figures usually show that about 85–90% of diabetics are type 2.

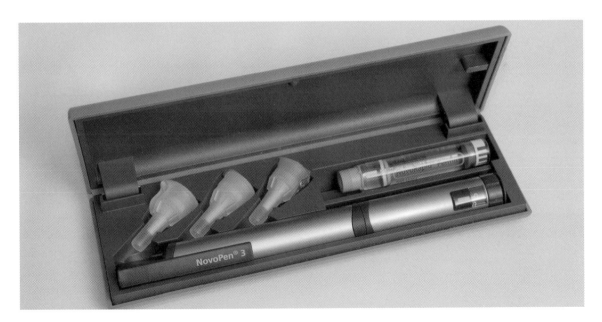

Figure 3.2 A typical insulin injection kit

The third category – which is relatively minor in comparison to the two main categories – is known as gestational diabetes mellitus (GDM) and occurs only in pregnant women (affecting about 3–10% of pregnancies). In most cases it is managed by diet and physical activity. GDM normally goes away once the baby is born, but it is important to understand that the condition can still cause an increased risk of future diabetes to mother and baby. For example, the American College of Sports Medicine (ACSM) has stated that approximately 50% of the women who develop gestational diabetes develop type 2 diabetes later in life, even though the reasons for this are not fully understood.

PREVALENCE

In the UK around 1.4 to 1.6 million people have been diagnosed with diabetes. But as type 2 diabetes often has few symptoms in the early stages, it is estimated that half of those with type 2 diabetes have not yet been diagnosed. The past 30 years have seen a threefold increase in the number of cases of childhood diabetes. Obesity levels have also risen dramatically, which has impacted on numbers of type 2 diabetics, as it is estimated that about 80% of type 2 diabetics are obese. Worldwide, it is estimated that in 2010 there were approximately 285 million people with type 2

diabetes (according to the report *Key Statistics on Diabetes*, published by Diabetes UK) and this figure is expected to increase to 438 million people by 2030. The report also includes the prevalence of diabetes in the adult population across the UK in 2009, which can be seen in table 3.1.

The impact of the extremely high numbers of the condition is evident in a 2007 report entitled *Diabetes in the NHS*, which states that the disease is costing the NHS an estimated £3.5 billion per annum (over £9 million each day), which equates to about 9% of the total NHS budget. Recently published work by the Yorkshire and Humber Public Health Observatory (2008) estimates that over 12% of all deaths in the 20- to 79-year-old category are as a result of diabetes, which suggests that prevention is vital. Even though the risk of diabetes increases as we age, it is thought that just over half of the forecast increase in diabetes cases between 2005 and 2010 will be attributable to the increase in overweight and obese people.

SYMPTOMS

There are many signs and symptoms associated with both types of diabetes. Table 3.2 presents a summary of common signs and symptoms.

Type 2 diabetes is also commonly associated with raised blood pressure, a disturbance of blood

Table 3.1	Prevalence of diabetes in the adult population in 2009	
Country	**Prevalence**	**Number of people**
England	5.1%	2,213,138
Northern Ireland	4.5%	65,066
Wales	4.6%	146,173
Scotland	3.9%	209,886

lipid (fat) levels and a tendency to develop thrombosis (blood clot). Because of these and other links, people with type 2 diabetes have an increased risk of coronary artery disease (leading to heart attacks, angina) peripheral artery disease (leg claudication, gangrene) and carotid artery disease (strokes, dementia). The long-term effects of diabetes can lead to many other conditions or complications. Such effects include:

- being the most common cause of blindness in people of working age;
- being the most common cause of amputation and end-stage kidney failure;
- increasing the likelihood of a stroke by four times;
- reducing life expectancy by 7–10 years for type 2 (15–20 years for type 1) and
- increasing the risk of heart disease by three to four times, and from depression by three times.

Some of these complications are as a result of poor blood flow and transport of nutrients around the body. This can also lead to nerve damage in about 60–70% of diabetics. This condition is known as 'neuropathy' and commonly causes a loss of sensation in the feet, known as 'diabetic foot'.

Diabetics can also suffer from 'retinopathy', which is the term used to describe damage to the retina.

DIAGNOSIS

Type 2 diabetes is difficult to diagnose as many people who have the disease show few or no symptoms and are often diagnosed accidentally following a routine medical examination or screening test for other conditions. Because of this, it is estimated that there are many thousands of people in the UK who are not aware that they have the condition. The majority of type 2 diabetics are usually diagnosed when other, often serious, health complications have occurred. Most diagnostic tests involve taking blood samples that measure glucose levels during certain conditions. There are three glucose tests (see pages 53–4) that are most commonly used: a random glucose test; a fasting glucose test; and a glucose tolerance test. A more accurate definition of how these tests are carried out can be found in the World Health Organization/International Diabetes Federation report 2006 (see the 'Recommended reading' at the end of this chapter for full details). This particular publication also shows the classifications

Table 3.2	Signs and symptoms of types 1 and 2 diabetes
Type 1	**Type 2**
Frequent peeing (polyuria)	Any type 1 symptoms
Unusual thirst (polydipsia)	Frequent infections
Extreme hunger (polyphagia)	Blurred vision
Unusual weight loss	Slow to heal cuts/bruises
Extreme fatigue, tiredness	Numbness in hands/feet
Irritability, mood changes	Recurring infections
Confused thinking	Incontinence in elderly
Vision problems	Often no symptoms

in relation to levels of blood glucose measured. Once a diagnosis of diabetes has been made by an appropriately qualified person (usually the GP), blood glucose levels are then sometimes monitored over a period of time so that the GP can be aware of any deterioration in the condition of an individual. When it comes to testing there are advantages and disadvantages, as with all forms of monitoring, in terms of time, expense and convenience, which is why it has been suggested that regular self blood glucose monitoring for people with type 2 diabetes can address some of these issues, as well as significantly improve quality of life and provide better blood sugar control. There are, however, some studies that contradict these suggestions so it remains an ongoing debatable topic. In terms of continued monitoring over a period of time, one of the standardised measurements of longer term blood glucose control is known as 'glycated haemoglobin' (HbA1c). The National Institute for Health and Clinical Excellence (NICE) guidelines recommend HbA1c measurements between two and six monthly (as decided by a qualified person) for people with type 2 diabetes, depending on stability of blood glucose control and changes in medication.

Interestingly, the American Indians would test for diabetes by seeing if ants were attracted to the urine of individuals. These days, however, for type 1 diabetes, a ketone test is usually carried out, which would only ever be done in a clinical environment. Ketones are chemicals in the body that are produced during the breakdown of fatty acids and are considered harmful at high levels. As insulin is used to regulate levels of ketones, it follows therefore that diabetics would suffer from high levels. A ketone test is done using a urine sample, usually at the following times:

- when the blood sugar is considered high;
- during an illness such as pneumonia, heart attack or stroke;
- when nausea or vomiting occur and
- during pregnancy.

There are also other tests for type 1 diabetes that can be done, known as 'antibody' tests. Carried out in a clinical environment, these tests include:

- glutamic acid decarboxylase (GAD) antibody tests;
- islet cell antibody (ICA) tests and
- insulin antibody tests.

RISK FACTORS

According to Diabetes UK, a person should ask their GP for a test for diabetes if they are white and over 40 years old, or if they are black, Asian or from a minority ethnic group and over 25 years old and have one or more of the following risk factors:

- a parent/sibling with diabetes
- a family background that is Alaska Native, American Indian, African American, Hispanic/ Latino, Asian American or Pacific Islander
- have had gestational diabetes or have given birth to a baby over 9 pounds
- have high blood pressure
- cholesterol levels are not in the normal range
- are physically inactive
- suffer from polycystic ovary syndrome (PCOS)
- have had impaired fasting glucose (IFG) or impaired glucose tolerance (IGT)
- have other clinical conditions associated with insulin intolerance
- have a history of cardiovascular disease.

TEST BOX: Blood glucose

Equipment needed

There are many blood glucose testing kits available, such as the Accu-Check® Aviva.

Random glucose test

This is where glucose levels are taken at a random time on two occasions. Any figure above 11.1 mmol/l is considered a diagnosis of diabetes.

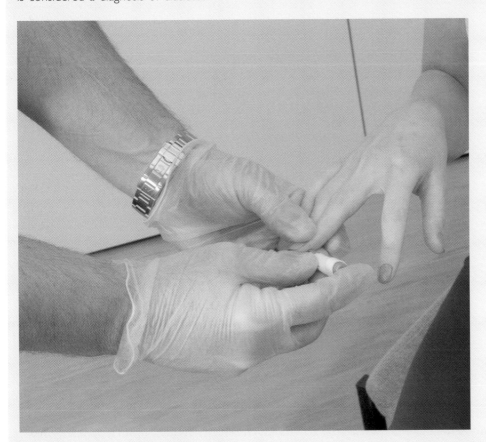

Figure 3.3 A typical blood glucose test

Fasting glucose test

This is where the glucose level is measured after an overnight fast and on two different days. Above 7.0 mmol/l is considered a diagnosis of diabetes. Table 3.3 overleaf shows the classification of blood level values for fasting glucose (mmol) per litre of blood.

Table 3.3	Fasting glucose test classification
Classification	**Blood glucose level (mmol/l)**
Good	4.4
Normal	less than 6.1
Impaired glucose (hyper)	6.1 to 7.0
Diabetes	more than 7.0
Hypoglycaemia	less than 2.8

Glucose tolerance test

This is where a glucose drink is given containing a standard amount of glucose (75 g). Blood samples are taken before the drink is given and 2 hours later. The test is done after an overnight fast. A 2-hour blood glucose level above 11.1 mmol/l is considered a diagnosis of diabetes. A level below 7.8 mmol/l is normal. If the level falls between these values, it suggests a decreased tolerance for glucose. This is known as impaired glucose tolerance (IGT). Impaired glucose tolerance is more than just a pre-diabetic state. People who have IGT are at increased risk of developing some of the conditions associated with diabetes, such as heart disease.

Physical inactivity is considered to be one of the main risk factors for the development of type 2 diabetes. Many studies, such as those by Kelley and Goodpaster (2001) and Ivy *et al.* (1999), show that type 2 diabetes is more common among people who are physically inactive. The link between inactivity and type 2 diabetes is further seen in studies such as those by Manson *et al.* (1991, 1992) and Lynch *et al.* (1996), which have suggested that people who take exercise have a 33–50% lower risk of developing type 2 diabetes, and that the greater amounts of exercise taken, the lower the risk of developing the disorder. Some studies have even looked at the type of activity that can reduce the risk. For example, a study by Hu and colleagues in 1999 showed that walking and cycling are associated with reduced risk of type 2 diabetes.

PHYSICAL ACTIVITY BENEFITS

If a diabetic person is under appropriate control prior to any activity, blood glucose concentration will decrease, and a lower insulin dosage may be required. It is important that the GP has given directions as to the correct dosages, which should be followed at all times otherwise problems could occur, as physical activity has an insulin-like effect. Physical activity is however, considered by many researchers to be of great importance in the care and treatment of diabetes. There are several benefits, which include those listed in table 3.4.

It should be noted, however, that many of the benefits of physical activity relate to type 2 diabetes and there is still uncertainty about the benefits related to type 1 diabetes. It is clear, though, that increasing physical activity levels before the onset of impaired glucose tolerance appears to have the

Table 3.4	Benefits of physical activity related to diabetics
Benefit	**Explanation**
Improved blood glucose control	Those with type 2 diabetes can use physical activity to help control blood glucose levels. Those with type 1 should not use this method for glucose control but use physical activity to gain other benefits.
Improved insulin sensitivity	As a result of improvements in insulin sensitivity a reduction in the insulin dose for type 1 diabetics may follow.
Fat loss	As weight loss can improve insulin sensitivity, this may lead to reductions in the insulin dose required by type 1 diabetics.
Cardiovascular benefits	These benefits can apply to those with diabetes as well as the healthy population.
Prevention of type 2 diabetes	Physical activity may play a role in the prevention of type 2 diabetes.

greatest potential for preventing type 2 diabetes. The level of physical activity related to the risk of diabetes has also been studied for many years. It is widely agreed that higher levels of physical activity are associated with lower risk of type 2 diabetes. In a study by Helmrich and colleagues (1991), different levels of energy expenditure (500-kcal increments) resulted in different risk levels for the development of type 2 diabetes (about a 6% decrease in risk for each increase in energy expenditure). Another study, by Hu *et al.* (1991), also reported that people who had higher levels of physical activity, such as walking and gardening, resulted in a lower risk of developing type 2 diabetes.

PHYSICAL ACTIVITY GUIDELINES

Most individuals with diabetes will be following management guidelines regarding medication, food intake, blood glucose levels and physical activity. Medications include glucose-lowering agents, antihypertensives, lipid-lowering agents, insulin and oral hypoglycemic agents (OHAs), which help the pancreas secrete more insulin and increase the sensitivity. As far as exercise guidelines are concerned, a study by Lynch *et al.* (1996) reported that moderate-intensity physical activities undertaken for at least one 40-minute session per week were needed to protect against the development of type 2 diabetes, while activity of lower intensity was not protective regardless of the duration. This should be viewed with caution, however, as it is widely agreed that there are many health-related benefits of undertaking a programme of regular lower-intensity physical activity even though the goal should be to increase the intensity when the individual is capable.

Generally speaking, activities that involve large muscle groups to a level of low-to-moderate intensity are recommended. Table 3.5 gives an overview of the general guidelines for physical activity for those individuals with diabetes.

In the event that an individual suffers from hypoglycaemia during an activity session it is

Table 3.5	Physical activity guidelines for diabetics	
	Aerobic training	**Strength training**
Mode	• Choose activities that can maximise caloric expenditure if obese	• Use an extended warm-up and gradual cool-down • Concentrate on upper body
Intensity	• Low to moderate intensity • 55–90%HRmax • 9–17 RPE	• Use loads within the individual's capability • Overload by increasing repetitions then intensity
Duration	• 5–30 minutes per session • Increase duration rather than intensity • Slow progression	• Perform 1 to 3 sets of 12–15 RM • 1–2 minutes' rest between exercises
Frequency	• 4–6 days per week	• 2–3 sessions per week • Encourage other forms of activity
Precautions	• Use appropriate footwear because of 'diabetic foot' • Monitor blood glucose frequently when initiating an exercise programme	• Exhale on greatest effort • Avoid impact or jarring activities • Try not to put too much pressure on the feet (squats etc.)

General precautions
- Make sure that the GP has given permission for physical activity.
- Training with someone is always advisable.
- Exercise caution when in hot weather and drink plenty of water at all times to avoid dehydration.
- Always carry fast-acting carbohydrate or glucose when doing activity.
- There is an increased risk of orthopaedic injury, cardiovascular disease and hyperthermia.
- Postpone activity if blood glucose >14.0 or <4.0 mmol/l, but check with GP to confirm latest figures.
- Try not to do activity late in the evening as hypoglycaemia can occur hours after intense activity.
- Try to do activities 1–2 hours after a meal.
- Symptoms such as confusion, nausea, vomiting, headache, coldness, tremors, etc. could indicate either hyper- or hypoglycaemia. Stop immediately and take appropriate action.
- Avoid activities that can increase blood pressure (such as overhead lifts) as this will increase the risk of retinopathy.

Table 3.6	Typical 10 g sources of glucose
Glucose source	**Amount**
Sugar	2 teaspoons or 3 sugar lumps
Honey	2 teaspoons
Dried fruit	¼ of a cup
Hypostop gel	Glucose 9.2 g/23 g oral ampoule
Milk	200 ml (about 1 cup)
Lucozade/sparkling glucose drinks	50–55 ml (non-diet versions)
Coca-Cola	90 ml (non-diet version)
Ribena original	15 ml (dilute with water)

Notes: ml = millilitres; g = grams

important to get that individual to take in glucose as quickly as possible. Approx 10 g of glucose is available from sources such as those shown in table 3.6. It is also advisable that, for every 30 minutes of activity, those with diabetes should also take about 10 g of glucose in order to avoid the onset of hypoglycaemia.

RECOMMENDED READING

American College of Sports Medicine (2009a) *ACSM's exercise management for persons with chronic diseases and disabilities* (3rd edn). Champaign, IL: Human Kinetics

American College of Sports Medicine (2009b) *ACSM's guidelines for exercise testing and prescription* (8th edn). London: Lippincott Williams & Wilkins

Armstrong, N. (2007) *Advances in sport and exercise science series: Paediatric exercise physiology*. Philadelphia, PA: Churchill Livingstone Elsevier, 326–331

Department of Health (2008) *Five years on delivery of diabetes national service framework*. London: DH Publications

Diabetes UK (2010) *Diabetes in the UK 2010: Key statistics on diabetes*. Available online at www.diabetes.org.uk

Farmer, A., Wade, A., Goyder, E., Yudkin, P., French, D., Craven, A., Holman, R., Kinmonth, A. & Neil, A. (2007) Impact of self monitoring of blood glucose in the management of patients with non-insulin treated diabetes: Open parallel group randomised trial. *British Medical Journal*, 335(7611): 132

Ford, E.S., Williamson, D.F. & Liu, S. (1997) Weight change and diabetes incidence. Findings from a national cohort of US adults. *American Journal of Epidemiology*, 146 (3): 214–222

Fox, C. & Kilvert, A. (2007) *Type 2 diabetes: Answers at your fingertips* (6th edn). London: Class Publishing

Harris, M. (2001) Frequency of blood glucose monitoring in relation to glycaemic control in patients with type 2 diabetes. *Diabetes Care*, 24: 979–982

Harris, M.I., Klein, R., Welborn, T.A. & Knuiman, M.W. (1992) Onset of NIDDM occurs at least 4–7 years before clinical diagnosis. *Diabetes Care*, 815–819

Hawley, J.A. & Zierath, J.R. (2008) Physical activity and type 2 diabetes. *Therapeutic effects and mechanisms of action*. Champaign, IL: Human Kinetics

Helmrich, S.P., Ragland, D.R., Leung, R. & Paffenbarger, R.S. (1991) Physical activity and reduced occurrence of non-insulin-dependent diabetes mellitus. *New England Journal of Medicine*, 325: 147–152

Hu, F.B., Sigal, R.J., Rich-Edwards, J.W., Colditz, G.A., Solomon, C.G., Willett, W.C., Speizer, F.E. & Manson, J.E. (1999) Walking compared with vigorous physical activity and risk of type 2 diabetes in women. *Journal of the American Medical Association*, 282: 1433–1439

Ivy, J.L., Zderic, T.W. & Fogt, D.L. (1999) Prevention and treatment of non-insulin-dependent diabetes mellitus. *Exercise and Sport Sciences Reviews*, 27: 1–35

Jaworska, J., Dziemidok, P., Kulik, T.B. & Rudnicka-Drozak, E. (2004) Frequency of self-monitoring and its effect on metabolic control in patients with type 2 diabetes. *Annales Universitatis Mariae Curie- Sklodowska-Sectio d – Medicina*, 59(1): 310–316

Kelley, D.E. & Goodpaster, B.H. (2001) Effects of exercise on glucose homeostasis in type 2 diabetes mellitus. *Medicine and Science in Sports and Exercise*, 33: S495–S501

Lynch, J., Helmrich, S.P., Lakka, T.A., Kaplan, G.A., Cohen, R.D., Salonen, R. & Salonen, J.T. (1996) Moderately intense physical activities and high levels of cardiorespiratory fitness reduce the risk of non-insulin-dependent diabetes mellitus in middle-aged men. *Archives of Internal Medicine*, 156: 1307–1314

Mackinnon, M. (1995) *Providing diabetes care in general practice* (2nd edn). London: Class Publishing

Manson, J.E., Nathan, D.M., Krolewski, A.S., Stampfer, M.J., Willett, W.C. & Hennekens, C.H. (1992) A prospective study of exercise and incidence of diabetes among USA male physicians. *Journal of the American Medical Association*, 268: 63–67

Manson, J.E., Rimm, E.B., Stampfer, M.J., Colditz, G.A., Willett, W.C., Krolewski, A.S., Rosner, B., Hennekens, C.H. & Speizer, F.E. (1991) Physical activity and incidence of non-insulin dependent diabetes mellitus in women. *Lancet*, 338: 774–778

McDowell, J.R.S. & Gordon, D. (1996) *Diabetes: Caring for patients in the community*. Edinburgh: Churchill Livingstone, 21–34

Murata, G.H., Duckworth, W.C., Shah, J.H., Wendel, C.S., Mohler, M.J. & Hoffman, R.M. (2009) Blood glucose monitoring is associated with better glycemic control in type 2 diabetes: A database study. *Journal of General International Medicine*, 24(1): 48–52

National Institute for Health and Clinical Excellence (NICE) (2002) *Inherited clinical guidance. Management of type 2 diabetes: Management of blood glucose*. London: NICE

National Institute for Health and Clinical Excellence (NICE) (2004) *Type 1 diabetes: Diagnosis and management of type 1 diabetes in children, young people and adults*. Clinical guideline 15. London: NICE

National Institute for Health and Clinical Excellence (NICE) (2008) *Type 2 diabetes: The management of type 2 diabete*s. Clinical guideline 66. London: NICE

National Statistics (2003) *Health Survey for England: Summary of key findings*. National Statistics (accessed 19 March 2010)

NHS (2007) *Diabetes in the NHS*. Available online at www.nhs.uk/conditions/diabetes/pages/introduction.aspx

NHS (2009) *Diabetes type I*. Available online at: www.nhs.uk/conditions/diabetes/pages/introduction.aspx. (last accessed 19th March 2010)

NHS Information Centre, Lifestyle Statistics (2009) *Statistics on obesity, physical activity and diet: England, February 2009*. London: NHS Information Centre for Health and Social Care

Overland, J.E., Hoskins, P.L., McGill, M.J. & Yue, D.K. (1993) Low literacy: A problem in diabetes education. *Diabetic Medicine*, 10(9): 847–850

Sudeck, C.D., Rubin, R.R. & Shump, C.S. (1997) *The Johns Hopkins guide to diabetes for today and tomorrow*. London: Johns Hopkins Press Ltd, 3–119

Valentine, V., Biermann, J. & Toohey, B. (2008) *Diabetes the new type 2. Your complete handbook for living healthfully with diabetes type 2*. New York: Penguin

World Health Organization/International Diabetes Federation (2006) *Definition and diagnosis of diabetes mellitus and intermediate hyperglycaemia. Report of a WHO/IDF consultation*. Geneva, Switzerland: WHO Press

Yorkshire and Humber Public Health Observatory (2008) *Diabetes attributable deaths. Estimating the excess deaths among people with diabetes*. YHPHO

USEFUL WEBSITES

Department of Health – www.dh.gov.uk

Diabetes UK – www.diabetes.org.uk

National Health Service – www.nhs.uk

National Institute for Health and Clinical Excellence – www.nice.org.uk

NHS Information Centre – www.ic.nhs.uk

World Health Organization – www.who.int/en

CHRONIC OBSTRUCTIVE PULMONARY DISEASE (COPD)

4

KEYPOINTS

- COPD is a life-threatening lung ailment that is not curable and will always be present in some way, however treatment can slow the progress of the disease.
- COPD is one of the most common respiratory diseases in the developed world, with an estimated 210 million who have the disease, and it is the fourth leading cause of death worldwide.
- There are approximately 900,000 people in England and Wales with COPD (and a possible further 450,000 undiagnosed).
- More than 250,000 people die each year at end stages of this condition.
- More than 3 million people died of COPD in 2005, which is equal to 5% of all deaths globally that year.
- The disease now affects men and women almost equally.
- Total deaths from COPD are projected to increase by more than 30% in the next 10 years.
- Even though physical activity will have no effect on the life expectancy of the sufferer there are many reported benefits that will have an effect on overall quality of life, such as:
  - reduction in symptoms;
  - improved muscular capacity;
  - increase in psychological benefits (reduction in anxiety, etc.);
  - improved ability for functional tasks and
  - lower risk of hospital admission and mortality.

WHAT IS IT?

Chronic obstructive pulmonary disease (COPD) is a life-threatening lung ailment that is often defined as 'a disease state characterised by persistent blockage of airflow that is not fully reversible'. In other words, the condition is preventable but not curable, and will always be present in some way; however, treatment can slow the progress of the disease. There are many respiratory conditions that can lead to COPD,

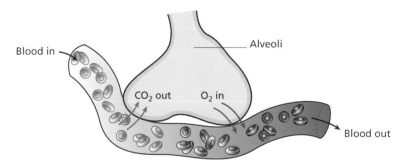

Figure 4.1 Oxygen and carbon dioxide exchange in the lungs

such as asthma (see chapter 5), emphysema and chronic bronchitis. It is widely agreed that smoking is the leading cause of COPD.

EMPHYSEMA

This particular condition that can lead to COPD is caused by damage to the alveoli (small air sacs) in the lungs. The alveoli in the lungs are responsible for the passage of oxygen (O_2) into the bloodstream and the passage of carbon dioxide (CO_2) out of the bloodstream, as illustrated in fig 4.1. This process of the two gases moving in and out is called 'gaseous exchange'. This is a simple process, which means that the oxygen we breathe in (part of the air) can be delivered to the bloodstream to be transported around the body. It also means that carbon dioxide, which is a waste product of energy production, can be breathed out. There are two main problems when damage to the alveoli occurs as a result of emphysema. First, the amount of oxygen that is delivered to the working muscles is much less, so those with emphysema will find it difficult to do any physical exertion. Second, alveoli are normally elastic but this is not the case in emphysema as they become hard and lose their elastic property. Because alveoli have lost their elastic recoil, breathing out becomes difficult, leading to trapped air in the lungs.

CHRONIC BRONCHITIS

This is also a condition that can lead to COPD. Chronic bronchitis occurs when the airways to the lungs (known as the bronchi) become inflamed with a build-up of mucus, leading to a chronic cough. Because of the inflammation and mucus build-up, the airways become narrowed, which reduces the amount of air in and out of the lungs. Just like emphysema, this can cause breathlessness with little or even no physical exertion.

PREVALENCE

According to the World Health Organization (WHO), COPD is one of the most common respiratory diseases in the developed world, and is considered to be the fourth leading cause of death worldwide (about 5% of all deaths are attributable to COPD). There are approximately 900,000 people in England and Wales with COPD (and a possible further 450,000 undiagnosed cases). The seriousness of the disease is illustrated by the fact that more than 250,000 people die each year at the end stages of the condition. The WHO has also published the following information in relation to COPD and its effects on a global scale.

- There are an estimated 210 million people who have COPD worldwide.
- More than 3 million people died of COPD in 2005, which is roughly equal to 5% of all deaths globally that year.
- The disease now affects men and women almost equally.
- Total deaths from COPD are projected to increase by more than 30% in the next 10 years.

SYMPTOMS

Even though there are many associated symptoms that are similar to those of other conditions, a list and description of the most common symptoms of COPD is shown in table 4.1. It is important to remember, however, that many of these listed symptoms can become worse over time. For example, daily activities such as walking up a short flight of stairs or carrying a suitcase can become very difficult as the condition gradually worsens over the years. For this reason, those with COPD are usually extremely deconditioned and they often find any form of physical activity very uncomfortable.

RISK FACTORS

Like most conditions, there are many recommended published sources that identify the risk factors for COPD. For this particular condition, however, there appears to be a general consensus relating to the symptoms, and little conflicting information. Table 4.2 gives an overview of the main risk factors that are common to a number of published sources, in particular those that were published by GOLD in 2008.

Table 4.1	Symptoms of COPD
Symptom	**Description**
Chronic cough	This can be mild but persistent
Chronic sputum production	This is where phlegm is brought up, usually by persistent coughing
Dyspnoea	This is breathlessness with even very slight exertion
Wheezing	Wheezing is commonly associated with COPD and gets worse with exercise
Repeat episodes of acute bronchitis	This will only be diagnosed by a GP
High blood CO_2	This will be in the form of muscle tremors, warm extremities and a bounding pulse
Low blood O_2	Restlessness, confusion and cyanosis (blue skin colour) are indications of low levels of oxygen in the blood
Muscle weakness	Muscle wasting occurs in about 30% of those with COPD
Exercise tolerance	Cardiovascular function is affected greatly by COPD

Table 4.2	Main risk factors for COPD
Genetic factors	It is thought that other factors (such as genetic), in addition to smoke exposure, are required for a person to develop COPD; even though most agree that there is a genetic link, what makes some individuals susceptible and others not to the effects of tobacco smoke is still unknown
Airway hyper responsiveness	Bronchial hyperresponsiveness (which is also a characteristic of asthma) is when people suffer sudden airway constriction in response to certain inhaled irritants; many people with COPD have this problem, but it is not known if the hyperresponsiveness is a cause or a consequence of COPD
Smoking	The main or primary cause of COPD is considered to be tobacco smoke (including second-hand or passive exposure); however, the likelihood of developing COPD increases with age and cumulative smoke exposure (greater number); at one time, COPD was more common in men, but the disease now affects men and women almost equally, according to the WHO
Occupational pollutants	Prolonged exposure to workplace dusts, chemicals and fumes has been linked to the development of COPD, even in non-smokers; the effect of occupational pollutants on the lungs appears to be substantially less than the effect of cigarette smoking
Dust, air pollution	Those individuals who live in large cities have a higher rate of COPD compared to those who live in rural areas; also, indoor air pollution from cooking and coal fires can be a contributory factor in COPD
Socio-economic status	According to the WHO, almost 90% of all COPD deaths in the world occur in low- and middle-income countries

RISK FACTORS

Like most conditions, there are many recommended published sources that identify the risk factors for COPD. For this particular condition, however, there appears to be a general consensus relating to the symptoms, and little conflicting information. Table 4.2 gives an overview of the main risk factors that are common to a number of published sources, in particular those that were published by GOLD in 2008.

DIAGNOSIS

The main problem for those with COPD is related to the function of the lungs, and in particular how efficient they are at getting oxygen in (to be used in energy production) and carbon dioxide (a waste product) out. There are several tests that are commonly used to measure lung function, or pulmonary function as it is also known. These tests are typically known as 'spirometry' tests and generally measure the rate at which the lungs change volume during forced breathing manoeuvres. Table 4.3 shows just some of the most common tests that are available for

Table 4.3	Common tests for respiratory conditions	
Measurement	**Units**	**Function**
Total lung capacity (TLC)	Litres	This is the total volume of air in the lungs at maximal inspiration (breathing in)
Forced vital capacity (FVC)	Litres	This is the maximum volume of air that can be exhaled (breathed out) with a maximal forced effort
Forced expiratory volume (FEV$_1$)	Litres	This is the volume of air forcefully expired in 1 second
Forced expiratory ratio (FER)	%	This is the relationship of FVC divided by FEV$_1$ and expressed as a percentage
Peak expiratory flow (PEF)	L/min-1	This simply refers to the maximum rate of airflow achieved during expiration
Maximal minute ventilation (MMV)	L/min-1	This is the maximum volume of air inhaled and exhaled in a predetermined time
Exercise-induced bronchoconstriction (EIB)	% increase or decrease	This is an indication of bronchoconstriction as a result of exercise

diagnosing many forms of respiratory conditions. The tests can also be used for tracking the progress of the various respiratory conditions (or the worsening in the case of COPD, as it is classed as a degenerative disease).

Individuals who are tested for suspected COPD (or asthma) often have to undergo measurements of forced vital capacity (FVC) and forced expiratory volume (FEV$_1$), which are both explained in the test box. These tests are usually done in a clinical environment by suitably qualified people, but they can also be done in a home or gym environment using equipment that is relatively inexpensive and easily obtained. If a diagnosis of COPD were being made in a clinical environment, before any testing took place, the individual being tested would normally be asked to take a bronchodilator (respiratory medication). After this was administered, a measurement of FVC and FEV$_1$ would be taken. A diagnosis would then normally be given using a combination of FEV$_1$ and FVC scores. For example, the measured FEV$_1$ score would then be compared to the individual's predicted value of FEV$_1$. If the FEV$_1$ score (measured in litres) was less than 80% of the predicted value for that individual, in combination with an FEV$_1$/FVC ratio (this is just FEV$_1$ divided by FVC) that was less than 70%, this would suggest the individual had a degree of COPD according to the percentage classifications given in table 4.4 (see page 65).

PREDICTING FEV^1

A predicted value of FEV$_1$ can be calculated quite simply by using a formula that requires only height (in metres) and age (calculate the age to a decimal place) to be measured. Note that there are different formulas for both males and females.

Test box: FEV$_1$ and FVC testing

Equipment needed
Spirometer (cost from £100), nose clip (optional, but helps), disinfectant wipes.

Test procedure
1 Have the subject take their normal bronchodilator if they use one.
2 Make certain that all equipment is sterilised – for example, mouthpiece. You can use disinfectant wipes for this.
3 Make sure that the subject is fully rested and fully informed about all the procedures they will undertake.
4 Place the nose clip on the subject.
5 Instruct the subject to take a maximal breath in and hold the breath momentarily.
6 Get the subject to place the mouthpiece of the spirometer in their mouth while still holding their breath (see fig 4.2).
7 Instruct the subject to breathe out forcefully, as hard and as fast as they can, until no air is left in the lungs.
8 Remove the mouthpiece and allow 15–30 seconds' rest before repeating the procedure.
9 Repeat until you achieve three measurements within 5% (or 100 ml) of each other.
10 Remove mouthpiece and nose clip, and disinfect them.

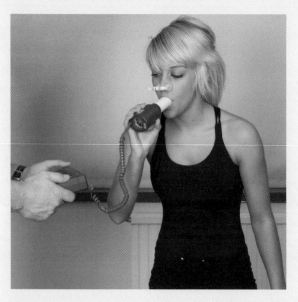

Figure 4.2 FEV$_1$ and FVC testing using a spirometer

> **Predicted FEV₁**
>
> Males: $FEV_1 = \{ (4.301 \times H) - (0.029 \times A) \} - 2.492$
>
> Females: $FEV_1 = \{ (3.953 \times H) - (0.025 \times A) \} - 2.604$
>
> Where H = height in metres, A = age in years

EXAMPLE DIAGNOSIS

Take the example of a 30-year-old female who is 1.6 m tall. This individual undergoes a spirometer test and scores 2.6 litres for her FEV_1. Her predicted FEV_1 is calculated using the prediction formula as follows:

$$Predicted\ FEV_1 = FEV_1 = \{ (3.953 \times H) - (0.025 \times A) \} - 2.604$$
$$= (3.953 \times 1.6) - (0.025 \times 30) - 2.604 = 2.9708\ litres$$

As 2.6 litres (the test score) is calculated to be 87.5% of her predicted score of 2.97 l, the female in the example would not be considered to have any particular respiratory problem as an FEV_1 test score that is above 80% of a predicted score would be classed as normal. Table 4.4 gives the full range of generally used classifications of percentage scores.

Even though diagnosis of COPD is always done by a suitably qualified person, the FVC and FEV_1 tests can also be used to monitor the progress of a particular individual who has already been diagnosed with the condition. It is important to note, however, that there is usually little or no improvement in lung function tests as a result of regular physical activity but at least the individual can be monitored to see if there is no more deterioration with the condition. This monitoring of progression (or not, as the case may be) can be done by taking a baseline measurement of FVC and FEV_1 before the start of any physical activity programme and then retaking the same measurements several times throughout the year to look for any change in the test results. The term forced vital capacity (FVC) is often defined as 'the maximum volume of air that can be expired after a full inspiration'. The term forced expiratory volume in 1 second (FEV_1) is often defined as 'the volume of air that can be forcibly exhaled from the lungs in the first second of a FVC measurement'. The testing procedure, therefore, is identical for both measurements; however, any individual must be instructed to focus on a hard and fast expiration during each test, while at the same time trying to exhale all air in the first second (making sure that the individual then continues to exhale as much air as possible to then get the FVC measurement). This type of testing can be done quickly and with little intrusion or embarrassment on the part of the individual. Testing is done using a device

Table 4.4	**Classification of predicted versus measured FEV₁**
FEV₁	**Interpretation**
>80% of predicted	Normal
66–80% of predicted	Mild obstruction
50–65% of predicted	Moderate obstruction
<50% of predicted	Severe obstruction

Table 4.5	Age- and gender-related normative values for forced vital capacity				
Age (yrs)	Male (cc)	Female (cc)	Age (yrs)	Male (cc)	Female (cc)
4	700	600	21	4320	2800
5	850	800	22	4300	2800
6	1070	980	23	4280	2790
7	1300	1150	24	4250	2780
8	1500	1350	25	4220	2770
9	1700	1550	26	4200	2760
10	1950	1740	27	4180	2740
11	2200	1950	28	4150	2720
12	2540	2150	29	4120	2710
13	2900	2350	30	4100	2700
14	3250	2480	31–35	3990	2640
15	3600	2700	36–40	3800	2520
16	3900	2700	41–45	3600	2390
17	4100	2750	46–50	3410	2250
18	4200	2800	51–55	3240	2160
19	4300	2800	56–60	3100	2060
20	4320	2800	61–65	2970	1960

Note: There are 1000 cc in 1 litre

known as a 'spirometer', which is a small hand-held instrument specifically designed for this purpose.

As with most tests of this nature, errors can sometimes occur during testing. One of the main errors is due to the subject not forcing all of the air completely out of the lungs. Another problem is that many subjects do not get a good seal around the mouthpiece and air leaks out when breathing.

FEV_1 and FVC can be analysed in different ways: either as a measured value or as a percentage of a predicted value, as shown previously when used for diagnosis purposes. As a simple measurement that can be used to monitor progression or for motivational purposes, FVC can also be classified by

age and gender. Table 4.5 shows scores for normal FVC where anything above this would be classed as being good and anything below not so good.

PHYSICAL ACTIVITY BENEFITS

Regular physical activity programmes can help many of those who have COPD, regardless of the severity of the condition. Even though physical activity will have no effect on the life expectancy of the individual, according to the GOLD report in 2008 there are many reported benefits that will have an effect on the overall quality of life, such as:

- reduction in symptoms;
- improved muscular capacity;
- increase in psychological benefits (reduction in anxiety, etc.);
- improved ability for functional tasks and
- lower risk of hospital admission and mortality.

There are many studies that show improvements in quality of life, as well as exercise capacity, exercise tolerance and muscular strength. Studies include those by Skumlien *et al.* (2007), Casaburi *et al.* (1997) and the GOLD report. It has also been shown (see Garcia-Aymerich *et al.*, 2006) that those people with COPD who undertake regular physical activity have a lower risk of being admitted to hospital with associated problems.

Table 4.6	Physical activity guidelines for mild COPD sufferers	
	Aerobic training	**Strength training**
Mode	• Ventilatory muscle training: 3–5 days per week, 30% of maximal inspiratory pressure, 30 minutes/day or typical aerobic activity; cycling in forward-lean position is advised	• Use a combination of free weights and body weight • Use functional activities such as standing to sitting squats or lifting tins on and off a shelf • Include mobility of the thoracic spine
Intensity	• 50% of peak oxygen uptake or maximal limits as tolerated by symptoms (3–4 on the dyspnoea scale)	• Use loads within the individual's capability • Overload by increasing intensity very slowly
Duration	• 5–30 minutes per session • Short bouts with rest periods are advised • Little progression is expected	• Perform 1 to 3 sets of 15–20 RM • Judge the repetitions more by fatigue
Frequency	• 3–5 days per week	• 2–3 days per week • Encourage other forms of exercise
Precautions	• Set intensity based on results of the walk test • Try to aim for higher intensity if possible	• Be aware that there is usually peripheral muscle weakness, especially in the arms

General precautions
- Moderate to severe COPD programmes should be done by a pulmonary rehabilitation team.
- There is usually a restricted range of upper body movement.
- Supervise all sessions.
- Stop activity if there is excessive breathlessness.
- Use inhaled medication if appropriate.

PHYSICAL ACTIVITY GUIDELINES

Regular physical activity programmes generally enhance the person's tolerance to physical activity, improve their quality of life and help to reduce their COPD symptoms. Even though there is usually no change to life expectancy, and little or no progression, it is important that those with COPD are encouraged to take up some form of physical activity. It is also important that those wishing to supervise physical activity of those with mild COPD clients inform the GP, as anyone with more than mild COPD will be under direct specialist supervision. For these individuals several types of programme may be prescribed, such as in-house, day outpatient clinics or home programmes. One form of activity that is generally recommended is that of ventilatory training (see chapter 5), even though the evidence to support it is lacking. It is thought that including this type of training as well as cardio training would benefit the individual more than just doing ventilator training on its own.

Table 4.7	Dyspnoea scale
Level	**Discomfort rating**
0	Nothing at all
0.5	Very, very slight
1	Very slight
2	Slight
3	Moderate
4	Somewhat severe
5	Severe
6	
7	Very severe
8	
9	Very, very severe
10	Maximal

As can be seen in the aerobic training guidelines in table 4.6, the use of a dyspnoea scale is recommended. This particular scale, as can be seen in table 4.7, is similar to a rating of perceived exertion (RPE) scale in that it gets the individual to rate their own level of discomfort. Those who are supervising physical activity for people with COPD should find this a useful tool as it gives immediate feedback from the individual doing the activity, which means that the intensity can be quickly adjusted without any delay or particular discomfort to the individual.

Many guidelines agree that extremes of temperature should be avoided with this population as those with the condition would find it difficult in both hot and cold environments. Those with more severe COPD will have very limited aerobic capacity, therefore several very short periods of activity with rest between should be encouraged. Regardless of the type of activity undertaken, a slow, progressive warm-up of gradual intensity should always take place. The primary goal is usually to begin with aerobic-type activity and then gradually introduce resistance-type activities. Individuals with COPD tend to become anxious during activity and hyperventilate, therefore slow, controlled breathing or pursed-lips breathing (see chapter 5) should be encouraged. The activity supervisor should be familiar with (and constantly monitor) warning signs of any cardiorespiratory problem such as worsening dyspnoea, swollen ankles and high resting heart rate, and if in any doubt cease any physical activity and seek medical advice.

RECOMMENDED READING

Agustí, A., MacNee, W., Donaldson, K. & Cosio, M. (2003) Hypothesis: Does COPD have an autoimmune component? *Thorax*, 58(10): 832–834

American College of Sports Medicine (2009a) *ACSM's exercise management for persons with chronic diseases and disabilities* (3rd edn). Champaign, IL: Human Kinetics

American College of Sports Medicine (2009b) *ACSM's guidelines for exercise testing and prescription* (8th edn). London: Lippincott Williams & Wilkins

Calverley, P.M. & Koulouris, N.G. (2005) Flow limitation and dynamic hyperinflation: Key concepts in modern respiratory physiology. *European Respiratory Journal*, 25(1): 186–199

Casaburi, R., Porszasz, J., Burns, M.R., Carithers, E.R., Chang, R.S. & Cooper, C.B. (1997) Physiologic benefits of exercise training in rehabilitation of patients with severe chronic obstructive pulmonary disease. *American Journal of Respiratory and Critical Care Medicine*, 155(5): 1541–1551

Celli, B.R., Cote, C.G., Marin, J.M., Casanova, C., Montes de Oca, M., Mendez, R.A., Pinto Plata, V. & Cabral, H.J. (2004) The body-mass index, airflow obstruction, dyspnea, and exercise capacity index in chronic obstructive pulmonary disease. *New England Journal of Medicine*, 350(10): 1005–1012

Devereux, G. (2006) ABC of chronic obstructive pulmonary disease. Definition, epidemiology and risk factors. *British Medical Journal*, 332(7550): 1142–1144

Fletcher, C. & Peto, R. (1997) The natural history of chronic airflow obstruction. *British Medical Journal*, 1: 1645–1648

Garcia-Aymerich, J., Lange, P., Benet, M., Schnohr, P. & Anto, J.M. (2006) Regular physical activity reduces hospital admission and mortality in chronic obstructive pulmonary disease: A population based cohort study. *Thorax*, 61(9): 772–778

GOLD (2008) *Global initiative for chronic obstructive lung disease. Pocket guide to COPD diagnosis, management and prevention: A guide for health care professionals.* Harbo, WA: Medical Communications Resources, Inc.

Halbert, R.J., Natoli, J.L., Gano, A., Badamgarav, E., Buist, A.S. & Mannino, D.M. (2006) Global burden of COPD: Systematic review and meta-analysis. *European Respiratory Journal*, 28(3): 523–532

Kumar, P. & Clark, M. (2005) *Clinical medicine* (6th edn). Edinburgh: Elsevier Saunders

Lacasse, Y., Goldstein, R., Lasserson, T.J. & Martin, S. (2006) Pulmonary rehabilitation for chronic obstructive pulmonary disease. *Cochrane Database of Systematic Reviews*, 4: CD 003793

Liesker, J.J., Wijkstra, P.J., Ten Hacken, N.H., Koëter, G.H., Postma, D.S. & Kerstjens, H.A. (2002) A systematic review of the effects of bronchodilators on exercise capacity in patients with COPD. *Chest*, 121(2): 597–608

Longmore, J.M., Wilkinson, I. & Rajagopalan, R.S (2004) *Oxford handbook of clinical medicine.* Oxford: Oxford University Press

Mahler, D.A. (2006) Mechanisms and measurement of dyspnea in chronic obstructive pulmonary disease. *Proceedings of the American Thoracic Society*, 3(3): 234–238

Mink, B.D. (1997) Exercise and chronic obstructive pulmonary disease: Modest fitness gains pay big dividends. *The Physician and Sports Medicine*, 25(11): 43–47

Murphy, T.F. (2006) The role of bacteria in airway inflammation in exacerbations of chronic obstructive pulmonary disease. *Current Opinion in Infectious Diseases*, 19: 225–230

National Institute for Health and Clinical Excellence (NICE) (2004) *Quick reference guide: COPD, management of chronic pulmonary disease in adults in primary and secondary care.* Clinical Guidelines 12. London: NICE

O'Donnell, D.E. (2006) Hyperinflation, dyspnea, and exercise intolerance in chronic obstructive pulmonary disease. *Proceedings of the American Thoracic Society*, 3(2): 180–184

Pauwels, R.A. & Rabe, K.F. (2004) Burden and clinical features of chronic obstructive pulmonary disease (COPD). *Lancet*, 364: 613–620

Puhan, M.A., Scharplatz, M., Troosters, T. & Steurer, J. (2005) Respiratory rehabilitation after acute exacerbation of COPD may reduce risk for readmission and mortality: A systematic review. *Respiratory Research*, 6: 54

Rennard, S.I. & Vestbo, J.R. (2006) COPD: The dangerous underestimate of 15%. *Lancet*, 367: 1216

Rosell, A., Monso, E., Soler, N., Torres, F., Angrill, J., Riise, G., Zalacain, R., Morera, J. & Torres, A. (2005) Microbiologic determinants of exacerbation in chronic obstructive pulmonary disease. *Archives of International Medicine*, 165: 891–897

Skumlien, S., Skogedal, E.A., Bjørtuft, Ø. & Ryg, M.S. (2007) Four weeks' intensive rehabilitation generates significant health effects in COPD patients. *Chronic Respiratory Disease*, 4(1): 5–13

World Health Organization (2000) *World health report. Health systems. Improving performance*. Geneva: WHO Press

World Health Organization (2009) WHO disease and injury country estimates. Available online at: http://www.who.int/healthinfo/global_burden_disease/estimates_country/en/index.html (accessed 11 June 2010)

Young, R.P., Hopkins, R.J., Christmas, T., Black, P.N., Metcalf, P. & Gamble, G.D. (2009) COPD prevalence is increased in lung cancer, independent of age, sex and smoking history. *European Respiratory Journal*, 34 (2): 380–386

USEFUL WEBSITES

American College of Sports Medicine – www.acsm.org

British Lung Foundation – www.lunguk.org

Global Initiative for Chronic Obstructive Lung Disease – www.goldcopd.org

National Institute for Health and Clinical Excellence – www.nice.org.uk

World Health Organization – www.who.int/en

5 ASTHMA

KEYPOINTS

- Asthma is a condition that can usually be reversed to some extent and is not always present, whereas COPD cannot be reversed.
- The causes of asthma can be broadly classified into two groups: exercise-induced asthma (EIA) or allergenic response.
- Approximately 80% of all asthmatics suffer from EIA.
- Severe asthma attacks are not responsive to standard treatments, which may in some circumstances lead to respiratory arrest and death.
- Approximately 5.2 million people (about 8% of the population) in the UK suffer from the effects of asthma (1 in 10 children and 1 in 20 adults).
- The highest reported prevalence globally is in Australia and New Zealand, with more than 15% of the population asthmatic.
- The lowest prevalence is in Africa and Asia, with between 5 and 10% of the population asthmatic.
- It is estimated that between 9 and 50% of winter athletes in the UK suffer from asthma, whereas summer athletes have the same percentage as the normal population.
- Benefits of exercise for those people with asthma are similar to the benefits of exercise for those with COPD, and include the following:
  - increased exercise endurance
  - increased functional status
  - decreased severity of reaction
  - improved quality of life.
- Physical activity can stimulate an asthma attack, even up to 4 hours later.

WHAT IS IT?

The term 'asthma' is derived from the Greek meaning 'to breathe hard', and is classed as a reversible obstructive airway disease that is caused as a result of several possible factors. Many people often confuse COPD (see chapter 4) with asthma, however the main difference is that asthma can usually be reversed to some extent and is not always present, whereas COPD cannot be reversed and those with COPD will always have the condition. The reversal of asthma can happen as a result of a particular treatment or sometimes without any obvious reason. Although asthma can develop in young people it may abate with maturity. In other words, it can get better in time to such an extent that it will not be noticeable. There are many possible reasons why people could develop respiratory conditions such as asthma. These include:

- possible genetic link through inherited genes (research continues);
- childhood exposure to allergens such as smoke, pollution and respiratory virus can increase risk and
- various triggers, including dust, infections, air pollutants, animals, drugs, pollen, smoke and certain chemicals (extrinsic) and exercise (intrinsic), can cause asthma attacks.

The causes of asthma can be broadly classified into two groups: as a result of either exercise (physical exertion) or as a result of an allergenic response. If the cause is as a result of exercise, it is otherwise known as 'exercise-induced asthma' (EIA) and if it is as a result of an allergenic reaction it is known as 'allergenic asthma'. Even though the symptoms of both categories are essentially the same, the causes are distinctly different. It should be noted however that there is a current research focus that is predicting that there is a greater genetic link than was first estimated.

Normal bronchiole

Asthmatic bronchiole

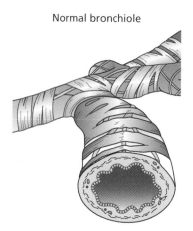 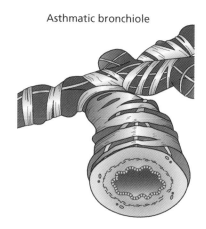

Figure 5.1 A normal and asthmatic airway (bronchiole)

ALLERGENIC ASTHMA

Various triggers, such as dust, chemicals and pet fur, are all potentially responsible for the onset of an asthma attack. During an allergic reaction, histamines are released from mast cells. Histamines are just hormones that have a powerful vasodilatation effect (they cause blood vessels to open wider) and mast cells are just cells where the histamines are stored. It is the reaction to the histamines that causes narrowing of the airways (the bronchi) to the lungs, which can quite quickly lead to breathing difficulties for the sufferer. Figure 5.1 shows the difference between a normal airway (bronchiole) and an airway that has constricted as a result of an asthmatic reaction.

EXERCISE-INDUCED ASTHMA (EIA)

This is where an asthma attack is brought on or stimulated by some form of physical exertion. Approximately 80% of all asthmatics suffer from EIA, which is also known as exercise-induced bronchoconstriction (EIB), as the airways leading to the lungs (bronchi) spasm and constrict as a result of any physical exertion. There are two distinct phases of an asthma attack that can occur as a result of partaking in physical activity. These are known as the 'early phase' and the 'late phase'. The early-phase asthma attack can occur between 5 and 20 minutes after the start of a physical activity session, and the late-phase asthma attack can occur up to 4 to 6 hours following the session. Even though the cause of the bronchoconstriction is not fully understood, at specific intensities of physical activity, cooling of the respiratory tract (airways) has been suggested (among other things) to be responsible for asthma attacks.

PREVALENCE

Figures published in 2005 by Asthma UK showed that approximately 5.2 million people (that is, about 8% of the population) in the UK suffer from the effects of asthma (1 in 10 children and 1 in 20 adults). Interestingly, the highest reported prevalence of asthma globally is in Australia and New Zealand, with more than 15% of the population asthmatic, and the lowest reported prevalence being in Africa and Asia, with between 5 and 10% of the population asthmatic. It is also interesting to note that between 9 and 50% of winter athletes in the UK have been diagnosed with asthma, whereas for summer athletes the percentage is the same as that for the normal population (about 8%).

SYMPTOMS

Those people with asthma typically experience shortness of breath (dyspnoea), laboured breathing accompanied by wheezing, constriction in the chest, and coughing or gasping, which is often worse at night or in response to physical exertion or even cold air. These common symptoms are normally referred to as an 'asthma attack', and can occur as a result of the narrowing of the airways caused by one or more of the following:

- involuntary contraction of the smooth muscle that surrounds the bronchi (airways leading to the lungs)
- swelling of the mucosal cells (cells producing a sticky substance called mucus) lining the inside of the bronchi

- excessive secretion of the mucosal cells lining the bronchi causing oedema (fluid build-up).

In relation to research on asthma, it has been suggested that the closing of the airways is the way that the body reacts to the perceived threat of the pollutants or allergens that actually cause the airways to swell. Unfortunately with this condition some of the more serious symptoms can be life threatening. For instance, during very severe attacks, a person with asthma can appear to turn blue (from a lack of oxygen in the blood), feel numbness in the limbs, have sweaty palms and can even lose consciousness. Some of the people who suffer the most severe asthma attacks are not always responsive to standard treatments (medication). If this is the case, the circumstances may even lead to respiratory arrest (where the breathing stops) and even death.

DIAGNOSIS

As discussed earlier, one of the main causes of asthma is a reaction to certain allergies (even though current research is suggesting genetics may be responsible). There are, however, a number of skin tests that can be carried out to determine which substances an individual may be allergic to. Generally speaking, most tests involve having a drop of the suspected allergenic solution placed on the forearm and then the skin being pricked with a small needle to allow the allergen into the bloodstream. If the individual is allergic to the particular substance, the skin will start to blister and will become itchy around that area. If this is the case, then it is recommended that the individual avoid that particular substance as it may contribute to an asthmatic reaction. The substances that are generally tested and considered to be very allergenic are extracts from pollen, house dust mite, cat and dog hair, and sometimes certain foods such as peanuts (a reaction to peanuts can be fatal in some cases). Also, as is generally the case with asthmatics, chest X-rays are carried out to check if there are any other conditions present that may be causing or making symptoms worse. In an individual with asthma there are often shadows on the X-rays caused by plugs of phlegm blocking the air passages. The plugs of phlegm could be present due to a reaction to certain mould spores. If the individual has an X-ray during a severe asthma attack, much of the lungs will show up black as there will be high levels of trapped air due to the restriction of breathing. In many cases, when diagnosing asthma, the GP or specialist will look for typical symptoms and signs, such as if an individual suffers from allergic conditions such as eczema or has a family history of asthma. With children, signs such as wheezing or a high-pitched sound when breathing out, recurrent wheezing, breathing difficulty, chest tightness, or a history of coughing that is worse at night, together with other information about the child, are often used in the diagnosis of asthma. In adults and older children, tests that look for airway restriction and function are sometimes used (see the list of tests in chapter 4, table 4.3). For example, there is a specific test known as an exercise-induced bronchoconstriction (EIB) test, which is commonly used for those individuals with suspected EIA. This particular test is used mainly in clinical environments to identify if there are any problems with breathing as a result of physical exertion. The test can also be used in non-clinical environments to monitor development of the condition.

EXERCISE-INDUCED BRONCHOCONSTRICTION TEST (EIB TEST)

The EIB test can be done quite easily and cheaply if there is access to a treadmill, heart rate monitor and spirometer. The test can provide both the tester and the individual being tested with valuable information such as knowing if and when to refer the individual being tested to a suitably qualified specialist. The procedure for an EIB test usually follows a relatively high-intensity (75 to 85% of maximal heart rate) period of exercise that lasts for a duration of at least 6 to 8 minutes, followed by a 15- to 20-minute period of rest. The guidelines in the test box show how lung or pulmonary function (FEV_1) before and after a bout of exercise should be compared, and how pulmonary function should be determined over a period of 15 to 20 minutes following the exercise bout (see chapter 4 for details of how to take FEV_1 measurements). The results of the test, once calculated or analysed, can then be classified as either mild, moderate or severe, according to typical published tables.

ANALYSING RESULTS

The purpose of analysing the results is to see if the subject has any form of bronchoconstriction as a result of doing exercise. This is done by measuring the percentage drop in FEV_1 where a drop of more than a certain percentage indicates some degree of bronchoconstriction. To do this, once you have a baseline FEV_1 measurement you can calculate each subsequent measurement as a percentage of that baseline measurement. Take the example of the female subject number 2 in table 5.1 (overleaf). The percentage drop between baseline and zero, baseline and 5, baseline and 10, and baseline and 15 all need to be calculated. This can then be added to the % column in table 5.1 (already done for you).

Test box: Exercise-induced bronchoconstriction (EIB)

Equipment needed
The cardiovascular exercise equipment to be used is the treadmill, plus spirometer and heart rate monitor.

Testing procedure
1   Calculate 50% and 75% of the subject's maximum predicted heart rate. This can be done simply by subtracting the subject's age from 220, which will give their predicted maximum heart rate, then calculating 50% and 75% of this.
2   Attach a heart rate monitor to the subject.
3   Take FEV_1 reading using a spirometer (as in fig 4.2) three times and record the maximum (write this score in the 'Base' (baseline) column in table 5.1).
4   Get the subject to exercise for 5 minutes at 50% of max and then for 8 minutes at 75% of max (as calculated earlier), adjusting the speed of the treadmill to suit.
5   At the end of the exercise, repeat the FEV_1 measurement immediately (write this score in the 'Zero L' column in table 5.1).

6 Sit the subject down and repeat FEV$_1$ measurements every 5 minutes, writing the score in the appropriate column in table 5.1 (5L, 10L, 15L).

7 Make sure you take three FEV$_1$ measurements each time and use the highest score.

Collection of results

When collecting the results of the EIB test, a simple method such as that in table 5.1 can be used, especially if testing more than one subject. Note, however, that information on sex, age, height and weight is always taken when testing.

Table 5.1				Example data collection table									
Subj.	Sex M/F	Age yrs	Height m	Weight kg	Base L	Zero L	%	5 L	%	10 L	%	15 L	%
1	F	36	1.54	56.2	4.8	4.9	100	4.6	96	4.2	87	4.2	87
2	F	31	1.64	64.3	4.4	4.2	95	3.5	79	3.0	68	3.2	72
3	M	27	1.83	86.7	5.6	5.5	98	5.1	91	5.3	95	5.4	96
4													
5													

Once the test is complete and all the data has been collected, the results can be analysed and also presented on a graph (such as that in fig 5.2). Presenting the results in graph form is useful as it gives a simple visual indication for both the tester and the subject to follow, especially as repeat tests can be done on the same graph. The results on the graph in fig 5.2 show the change in FEV$_1$ readings from baseline up to 15 minutes after exercise for all three subjects. Note that the data in the % columns are explained in the section: 'Analysing results'.

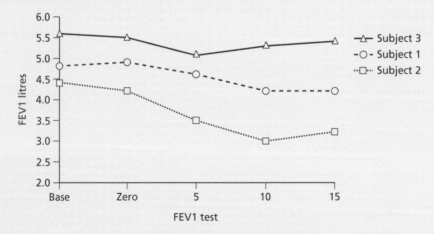

Figure 5.2 Graph to show results of FEV$_1$ bronchoconstriction test for three subjects

Example for subject 2 if the baseline FEV₁ is 4.4 litres

Baseline to zero minute % drop:
4.2 divided by 4.4 = 0.95 then multiply this by 100 to give a percentage = 95%

Baseline to 5 minute % drop:
3.4 divided by 4.4 = 0.79 then multiply this by 100 to give a percentage = 79%

Baseline to 10 minute % drop:
3.0 divided by 4.4 = 0.68 then multiply this by 100 to give a percentage = 68%

Baseline to 15 minute % drop:
3.2 divided by 4.4 = 0.72 then multiply this by 100 to give a percentage = 72%

Table 5.2	Classification of bronchoconstriction
Classification	**Measurement**
Mild	10–24% fall in FEV_1
Moderate	25–39% fall in FEV_1
Severe	40% or greater fall in FEV_1

As can be seen in the example, the FEV_1 at zero has dropped by 5% to 95% of the baseline result. The FEV_1 at 5 minutes then drops to 79% of the baseline, at 10 minutes drops to 68% and then at 15 minutes rises slightly to 72%. Once the percentage drops have been calculated in this way, table 5.2 can then be used to classify the extent, if any, of the bronchoconstriction. Subject 2 in the example dropped by a maximum of 32% at the 10-minute measurement so, according to the classifications in table 5.2, subject 2 clearly has moderate bronchoconstriction. Subject 3 has borderline mild bronchoconstriction with a maximum drop of only 9%, whereas subject 1 is classed as mild with a maximum 13% drop. If the percentage falls more than 10% of the baseline measurement it will indicate a certain amount of bronchoconstriction, but be aware that the percentage change can go up as well as down.

RISK FACTORS

Like all risk factors, the ones for asthma include those that are considered modifiable (something can be done to reduce the risk) and those that are considered non-modifiable. For example, gender is a risk factor for asthma that is non-modifiable but, as can be seen in table 5.3 (overleaf), asthma shows a predisposition to female rather than male, especially when related to morbidity. Even though there is an abundance of research that is currently investigating potential genetic links associated with asthma, there is obviously nothing that can be done about this particular risk factor in terms of programme modification. Table 5.3 gives a description of some of the modifiable risk factors for this condition.

PHYSICAL ACTIVITY BENEFITS

Physical activity has often been shown to be a key component in the rehabilitation of individuals with respiratory disease such as asthma. Research carried out by the European Respiratory Society in 1992 suggests that the benefits of physical activity for those people with asthma are similar to

Table 5.3	Risk factors for asthma
Risk factor	**Comment**
Allergies	• A positive skin test for allergies in children between the ages of 3–14
	• In adults, the more positive reactions to allergens in a skin test, the higher the odds of having asthma
Home circumstances	• Exposure to certain allergens in infancy and early childhood with exposure to cigarette smoke being the main problem
BMI	• In the UK and USA, the rise in asthma prevalence has mirrored the rise in the prevalence of obesity
Socio-economic status	• The incidence of asthma is highest among low-income populations, both nationally and worldwide
	• Asthma deaths are most common in those low-income neighbourhoods whose populations consist of large percentages of ethnic minorities
Gender	• Even though this is a non-modifiable risk factor, women account for nearly 65% of all asthma-related deaths

the benefits for those with COPD, and include the following:

• increased exercise endurance
• increased functional status
• decreased severity of reaction
• improved quality of life.

An important factor to remember, however, is that improvement as a result of physical activity can be expected regardless of the severity of the disease. For this reason, physical activity should always be part of a lifestyle routine for all asthmatics no matter what their age or how severe the condition is.

PHYSICAL ACTIVITY GUIDELINES

For those asthmatics who are not used to physical activity, emphasis should be placed on long, gradual warm-ups where the intensity of the activity is slowly increased. The main aerobic activity should be kept at a relatively low level until the individual becomes accustomed to the level. This may take several months, but slow progression is the key. There are many sources of advice relating to physical activity for asthmatics. Table 5.4 gives an overview of the more recent published advice that is separated into specific and general categories.

VENTILATORY MUSCLE TRAINING

This is a procedure that involves using a breathing device that adds resistance when an individual breathes through it. A device like this is often given to an individual who has moderate to severe asthma by a specialist, who will also give advice on how to use the device.

IN CASE OF AN ASTHMA ATTACK ...

It is possible that an individual may develop an asthma attack as a result of participating in some

Table 5.4	Physical activity guidelines for asthmatics	
	Aerobic training	**Strength training**
Mode	• Ventilatory muscle training: 3–5 days per week, 30% of maximal inspiratory pressure, 30 minutes/day or typical aerobic activity	• Use an extended warm-up and gradual cool-down • Concentrate on upper body
Intensity	• 50% of peak oxygen uptake or maximal limits as tolerated by symptoms (3–4 on the dyspnoea scale)	• Use loads within the individual's capability • Overload by increasing repetitions then intensity
Duration	• 5–30 minutes per session. • Increase duration rather than intensity • Slow progression	• Perform 1 to 3 sets of 12–15 RM • 1–2 minutes' rest between exercises
Frequency	• 3–5 days per week	• 2–3 sessions per week • Encourage other forms of exercise
Precautions	• Pursed-lips breathing – in through nose and out through pursed lips twice as long	• Exhale on greatest effort

General precautions

- An inhaler should be carried.
- As with diabetics, training with someone is always advisable.
- Take medical advice; the asthmatic should follow a medication plan to prevent EIA.
- There should be thorough screening to identify causes of asthma.
- Running causes more attacks than cycling and walking; the fewest attacks happen with swimming (the air above the water tends to be warmer and contains more moisture).
- In cold weather a scarf or face mask can be used to trap moisture.
- Be aware of social implications (coughing and sputum clearance).

form of physical activity. Even though the risk of an asthmatic event cannot be eliminated entirely by following the physical activity precautions given in table 5.4, it is important that steps should be taken in the event of an asthma attack occurring. Even though an asthma attack could be moderate, severe or life threatening, it is best to treat it as severe until it is established that it is not. It would also make sense to check that any individual who has been diagnosed as asthmatic should be made aware of these steps even though they will probably have a more extensive knowledge of the condition.

In the event of an asthma attack

STEP 1: Make the subject comfortable and calm them.

STEP 2: Have the subject focus on breathing.

STEP 3: Use pursed-lips breathing technique.

STEP 4: If no improvement, call for help.

If the person supervising the activity does attend to an individual who has had an asthma attack and emergency services are required, they must stay with the individual until help arrives. They must also continue to make the individual as comfortable and as calm as possible, and keep them using the pursed-lips breathing technique.

RECOMMENDED READING

American College of Sports Medicine (2009a) *ACSM's exercise management for persons with chronic diseases and disabilities* (3rd edn). Champaign, IL: Human Kinetics

American College of Sports Medicine (2009b) *ACSM's guidelines for exercise testing and prescription* (8th edn). London: Lippincott Williams & Wilkins

Ayres, J. (1999) *Family doctor guide to asthma*. London: Dorling Kindersley

Barbee, R.A. & Murphy, S. (1998) The national history of asthma. *Journal of Allergy Clinical Immunology*, 102: 65–72

Barnes, J. & Newhouse, M.T. (1991) *Conquering asthma: An illustrated guide to understanding and self care for adults and children*. Hamilton, Ontario: Manson Publishing

Barnes, J., Rodger, W. & Thomson, N.C. (1998) *Asthma basic mechanics and clinical management* (3rd edn). London: Academic Press

Boner, A.L. & Martinati, L.C. (1997) Diagnosis of asthma in children and adolescents. *European Respiratory Review*, 7(40): 2–7

Bundgaard, A. (1991) Exercise-induced asthma. *Primary Care*, 18(4): 809–891

Carlsen, K.H., Engh, G., Mork, M. & Schroder, E. (1998) Cold air and exercise-induced bronchoconstriction in relationship to metacholine bronchial responsiveness: Different patterns in asthmatic children and children with other chronic lung diseases. *Respiratory Medicine*, 92(2): 308–315

Celedon, J.C., Litonjua, A.A., Ryan, L., Platts-Mills, T., Weiss, S.T. & Gold, D.R. (2002) Exposure to cat allergen, maternal history of asthma, and wheezing in first 5 years of life. *Lancet*, 360: 781–782

Christensen, P., Thomasen, S.F., Rasmussen, N. & Backer, V. (2007) Exercise-induced inspiratory stridor. An important differential diagnosis of exercise-induced asthma. *Ugeskr Laeger*, 169(47): 4047–4050

Chung, K.F. (2002) *Clinicians' guide to asthma*. London: Arnold, Hodder Headline Group

Clark, C.J. & Cochrane, L.M. (1999) Physical activity and asthma. *Current Opinion in Pulmonary Medicine*, 5(1): 68–75

Ehrman, K.J., Gordon, M.P., Visich, S.P. & Keteyian, J.S. (2003) *Clinical exercise physiology*. Champaign, IL: Human Kinetics

Fanta, C.H. (2009) Asthma. *New England Journal of Medicine*, 360(10): 1002–1014

Fowler, M., Davenport, M. & Garg, R. (1992) School functioning of US children with asthma. *United States: Paediatrics*, 939–944

Freeman, C.G., Schneider, D. & McGarvey, P. (2003) The relationship of health insurance to the diagnosis and management of asthma and respiratory problems in children in a predominantly Hispanic urban community. *American Journal of Public Health*, 93(8): 1316–1319

GOLD (2008) *Global initiative for chronic obstructive lung disease. Pocket guide to COPD diagnosis, management and prevention: A guide for health care professionals*. Harbor, WA: Medical Communications Resources, Inc.

Gold, D.R. & Wright, R. (2005) Population disparities in asthma. *Annual Review of Public Health*, 26: 89–113

Hargreave, F.E. & Parameswaran, K. (2006) Asthma, COPD and bronchitis are just components of airway disease. *European Respiratory Journal*, 28(2): 264–267

Holgate, S.T. & Pauwels, R.A. (1999) *Asthma: Fast facts indispensable guide to clinical practice*. Oxford: Health Press Limited

International Study of Asthma and Allergies in Childhood (ISAAC) Steering Committee (1998) Worldwide variation in prevalence of symptoms of asthma, allergic rhino conjunctivitis, and atopic eczema. *Lancet*, 351: 1225–1232

Jaakkola, J.K., Parise, H., Kislitsin, V., Lebedeva, N.I. & Spengler, J.D. (2004) Asthma, wheezing, and allergies in Russian schoolchildren in relation to new surface materials in the home. *American Journal of Public Health*, 94(4): 560–562

Lane, D.J. (1996) *Asthma the facts* (3rd edn). Oxford: Oxford University Press

Leutholtz, B.C. & Ripolli, I. (2000) *Exercise and disease management.* London: CRC Press

Levy, M. (2006) The efficiency of asthma case management in an urban school district in reducing school absences and hospitalizations for asthma. *Journal of School Health*, 76(6): 320–325

Levy, M., Hilton, S. & Barnes, G. (2000) *Asthma at your fingertips* (3rd edn). London: Class Publishing

Lewis, J. (1995) *The asthma handbook: A definitive guide to the causes, symptoms and all the latest treatments.* London: Vermilion

Magnus, P. & Jaakkola, J.J. (1997) Secular trend in the occurrence of asthma among young adults: Critical appraisal of repeated cross sectional surveys. *British Medical Journal*, 314: 1795–1799

Naqvi, M., Thyne, S., Choudhry, S., Tsai, H.J., Navarro, D., Castro, R.A., Nazario, S., Rodriguez-Santana, J.R., Casal, J., Torres, A., Chapela, R., Watson, H.G., Meade, K., LeNoir, M., Avila, P.C., Rodriguez-Cintron, W. & Burchard, E.G. (2007) Ethnic-specific differences in bronchodilator responsiveness among African Americans, Puerto Ricans, and Mexicans with asthma. *Journal of Asthma*, 44(8): 639–648

National Asthma Campaign (2001) Out in the open: A true picture of asthma in the United Kingdom today. *Asthma Journal*, 6: 3–14

National Asthma Education and Prevention Program (1997) *Expert panel report: Guidelines for the diagnosis and management of asthma.* National Institutes of Health. Bethesda, MD: US Department of Health, 97–4051

Ober, C. & Hoffjan, S. (2006) Asthma genetics 2006: The long and winding road to gene discovery. *Genes and Immunity*, 7(2): 95–100

Paules, R. (1996) The current place of nedocromil sodium in the treatment of asthma. *Journal of Allergy and Clinical Immunology*, 98(5): 151–156

Pauwels, R.A., Lofdahl, C.G., Pride, N.B., Postma, D.S., Laitinen, L.A. & Ohlsson, S.V. (1992) European Respiratory Society study on chronic obstructive pulmonary disease (EUROSCOP): Hypothesis and design. *European Respiratory Journal*, 5: 1254–1261

Pearlman, D.S., Rees, W., Schaefer, K., Huang, H. & Andrews, W.T. (2007) An evaluation of Levalbuterol HFA in the prevention of exercise-induced bronchospasm. *Asthma Journal*, 44(9): 729–733

Peat, J.K., Tovey, E., Toelle, B.G., Haby, M.M., Gray, E.L., Mahmic, A. & Woolcock, A.J. (1996) House dust mite allergens: A major risk factor for childhood asthma in Australia. *American Journal of Respiratory and Critical Care Medicine*, 153: 141–146

Randolph, C. (2007) Exercise-induced bronchospasm in children. *Clinical Review of Allergy Immunology*, 34(2): 205–216

Salam, M., Islam, T. & Gilliland, F.D. (2008) Recent evidence for adverse effects of residential proximity to traffic sources on asthma. *Current Opinion in Pulmonary Medicine*, 14(1): 3–8

Von Mutius, E. (1996) Progression of allergy and asthma through childhood to adolescence. *Thorax*, 51(1): 3–6

Von Mutius, E., Martinez, F.D., Fritzsch, C., Nicolai, T., Roell, G. & Thiemann, H.H. (1992) Prevalence of asthma and atopy in two areas of West and East Germany. *American Journal of Respiratory and Critical Care Medicine*, 149: 358–364

Wardlaw, A.J. (1993) *Asthma.* Oxford: BIOS Scientific Publishers Limited

USEFUL WEBSITES

American College of Sports Medicine – www.acsm.org

Asthma News in the UK and Ireland – www.asthma-uk.co.uk/index.htm

Asthma UK – www.asthma.org.uk

British Lung Foundation – www.lunguk.org

Global Initiative for Chronic Obstructive Lung Disease – www.goldcopd.org

National Institute for Health and Clinical Excellence – www.nice.org.uk

World Health Organization – www.who.int/en

// **HYPERTENSION**

6

KEYPOINTS

- The term 'hypertension' simply means high blood pressure, whereas 'hypotension' means low blood pressure.
- Hypertension increases the risk of cardiovascular disease, stroke, peripheral vascular disease and kidney failure.
- Around 11% of all disease burden in developed countries is due to raised blood pressure, and over 50% of coronary heart disease and almost 75% of stroke in developed countries is due to high systolic blood pressure levels.
- It is estimated that 22% of heart attacks in western Europe and 25% of heart attacks in central and eastern Europe are due to a history of high blood pressure.
- 31% of men and 29% of women have high blood pressure (at least 140 mmHg systolic and/or 90 mmHg diastolic blood pressure and/or on treatment for hypertension) and more than half of over-65s in England suffer from hypertension.
- High blood pressure has resulted in 62,000 unnecessary deaths every year.
- The mean systolic blood pressure is 131.4 mmHg in men and 125.9 in women, and the mean diastolic blood pressure is 74.3 mmHg in men and 73.2 in women.
- It is estimated that 14% of deaths from coronary heart disease in men and 12% in women are due to raised blood pressure, and that reducing the proportion of the population with high systolic blood pressure (140 mmHg) by 50% would prevent more than 18,000 coronary heart disease events in England alone.
- Regular physical activity may lead to an average reduction of 8–10 mmHg for systolic pressure and up to 7–8 mmHg for diastolic pressure.
- Some studies have actually shown a reduction in blood pressure in subjects up to the age of almost 90 years.

WHAT IS IT?

The term 'hypertension' simply refers to high blood pressure, whereas 'hypotension' refers to low blood pressure. When the term blood pressure is used it actually refers to the pressure of the blood against the walls of the arteries it flows through. This is why arteries have thick walls compared to veins, as there is much more pressure in them. The medical definition of high blood pressure often refers to a condition in which blood pressure is chronically elevated above levels that are considered desirable. Hypertension is without doubt a major health problem in which the risk of cardiovascular disease, stroke, peripheral vascular disease and kidney failure is increased with increases in blood pressure. The amount of pressure that the blood exerts on the artery walls is determined by 'cardiac output' (CO) and 'total peripheral resistance' (TPR). CO is the total amount of blood pumped out of the heart every minute, and TPR refers to the combined pressure on all of the artery walls due to the flow of blood through them. When blood pressure is measured using an instrument known as a sphygmomanometer, there are two readings that are recorded. One is the systolic pressure and the other is the diastolic pressure; both are measured in millimetres of mercury (mmHg). The pressure increases when blood flows as the heart contracts, and then decreases as the heart is filling up and not contracting.

It is easier to think of hypertension as having two main classification groups: essential and secondary. Essential hypertension is the most prevalent hypertension type, affecting about 90–95% of hypertensive patients. With this particular classification, although no direct cause can be identified, there are many factors (covered in this chapter) that can increase the risk of developing hypertension. Secondary hypertension, on the other hand, is slightly different in that it results from an identifiable cause such as kidney disease. The main difference is that secondary hypertension is usually addressed by treating the underlying cause of the elevated blood pressure.

> **Systolic:** This is the pressure on the artery walls when the heart is in a state of contraction (known as systole).
>
> **Diastolic:** This is the measurement on the artery walls when the heart is in a state of relaxation (known as diastole).

PREVALENCE

The World Health Report of 2002 estimates that around 11% of all disease burden in developed countries is due to raised blood pressure, and that over 50% of coronary heart disease (CHD) and almost 75% of stroke in developed countries is due to high systolic blood pressure levels. In 2004, the INTERHEART study published in the *Lancet* estimated that 22% of heart attacks in western Europe and 25% of heart attacks in central and eastern Europe were due to a history of high blood pressure, and that those with a history of hypertension were at just under twice the risk of a heart attack compared to those with no history of hypertension. According to the *Health Survey for England* in 2007, 31% of men and 29% of women had high blood pressure (at least 140 mmHg systolic and/or 90 mmHg diastolic blood pressure and/or on treatment for hypertension) and more than half of over-65s in England suffer from hypertension. High blood pressure was found to be rare below the age of 35 years, but increased with age in both men and women. Up to the age of 64 years, it was higher among men than women, and by the age of 75 and over it was higher among women than men. The survey also showed that 46% of men and 53% of women were taking medication to treat the condition (the treatment rate increased with age). In England the average systolic blood pressure is estimated to be 131.4 mmHg in men and 125.9 in women, and the average diastolic blood pressure is 74.3 mmHg in men and 73.2 in women. As a consequence, high blood pressure has resulted in 62,000 unnecessary deaths every year. Hypertension is linked to coronary heart disease, which kills more than 70,000 people in England every year. It is estimated that 14% of deaths from CHD in men and 12% in women are due to raised blood pressure and that reducing the proportion of the population with high systolic blood pressure (140 mmHg) by 50% would prevent more than 18,000 coronary heart disease events in England alone.

SYMPTOMS

Hypertension is known as the 'silent killer' because it can cause considerable damage to the blood vessels, heart, brain and kidneys before it causes any pain or shows any noticeable symptoms.

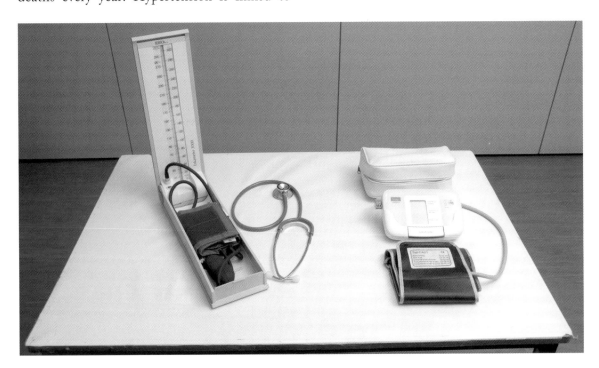

Figure 6.1 Typical manual mercury and automatic sphygmomanometer

DIAGNOSIS

Blood pressure is usually measured at the left brachial artery (the main artery in the upper arm) while the subject is normally seated or lying down using a device called a sphygmomanometer (see fig 6.1). Taking blood pressure in this way is known as 'auscultatory' measurement.

There are several types of sphygmomanometer that can be used, such as the manual mercury, manual aneroid and automatic electrical. The manual mercury sphygmomanometer is considered to be more accurate than the other types, but the risk of mercury has prompted many countries to ban their use in favour of the aneroid-type device. An accurate device is absolutely essential for all blood pressure measurements because if the device used is inaccurate, then the measurement taken is of little use. Even though some manufacturers make claims regarding the accuracy of their devices, independent information can be obtained from websites such as those of the European Society of Hypertension (ESH) or the British Hypertension Society (BHS). The measurement of blood pressure is not a straightforward process as blood pressure can be affected by many factors, such as those listed in table 6.1.

Table 6.1	Factors affecting blood pressure
Factor	**Comment**
Anxiety	This is often called the 'fight or flight' phenomenon, and can raise blood pressure by as much as 30 mmHg or more; those people who are anxious can see blood pressure fluctuate during the day by as much as 50–60 mmHg for systolic blood pressure
White-coat effect	An increase in blood pressure often occurs in hospitals or doctors' surgeries when patients are frightened or anxious
White-coat hypertension	People with normal blood pressure can become hypertensive during repeated clinic blood pressure measurements, but pressures then settle to normal outside the medical environment
Arm support	If the arm in which measurement is being made is unsupported, increasing blood pressure and heart rate can result; diastolic blood pressure may be increased by as much as 10%; it is essential, therefore, for the arm to be supported during blood pressure measurement, especially when the individual is in the standing position
Arm position	If the arm is below heart level during measurement this can lead to an overestimation of systolic and diastolic pressures; the magnitude of this error can be as great as 10 mmHg for systolic and diastolic readings; for this reason, the forearm must always be at the level of the heart during measurements
Which arm?	Blood pressure can be different in each arm; clinicians often take measurements on both arms on the first consultation and, if the difference is greater than 20 mmHg for systolic or 10 mmHg for diastolic pressure, further evaluation is done
Other factors	Many other factors, such as exercise, eating, smoking, alcohol, temperature, illness and pain, can all affect blood pressure

Some factors only have a small effect, but others can affect blood pressure quite substantially. Even though it is not always possible to eliminate all these factors, the tester should at least try to address them when taking blood pressure measurements. For instance, follow the simple pre-measurement guidelines listed below.

- Make sure that the individual is relaxed in a quiet and private room for at least 5 minutes before taking the measurement to try to alleviate any stress or anxiety. Advise individuals to avoid caffeine and nicotine for 30 minutes before the measurement as these can raise blood pressure.
- Empty the bladder as a full bladder can also elevate blood pressure.
- Make sure that the individual is seated with their legs and back supported.

TAKING BLOOD PRESSURE

There are many sources of information relating to the manual measurement of blood pressure, such as Beevers *et al.* (2001). However, most sources are similar in their direction so that standardisation of measurement can be achieved. Typical instructions relating to the placement of the manual device, the taking of the measurement and the interpretation of the sounds can be seen in the test box. Measuring blood pressure levels in older people can be more difficult than in younger people as, in general, older people have a greater blood pressure variability, therefore it is important that more than one measurement is taken on several different occasions just to make sure that the readings are fairly consistent. It is also common

that both sitting and standing measurements are taken in this age group.

The various auscultatory sounds associated with the different phases of the measurement are often difficult to detect but are described in table 6.2. You will notice, however, that there is something called an 'auscultatory gap'. This is the name given when the sounds disappear altogether for a short period of time following phase II. This only occurs sometimes with certain people when taking blood pressure measurements, which is why it is important to try to find the starting pressure as described in the test box just in case there is an auscultatory gap that leads to phase III being mistaken for phase I.

A clinical diagnosis of hypertension is never done using one measurement only and should be done only by a suitably qualified individual. The decision is normally based on an average of two or more readings measured during each of two or more visits following an initial screening procedure. Blood pressure classifications can differ depending on the source. However, the figures in table 6.3 show the ranges of systolic and diastolic classifications, which are in units of mmHg as recommended by the American College of Sports Medicine (ACSM). It is important to note that only one of the blood pressure readings (systolic pressure or diastolic pressure) needs to be high in order for the subject to be classed in the appropriate hypertensive range. For example, if an individual had a systolic pressure reading of 118 mmHg and a diastolic pressure reading of 92 mmHg, then they would be classed (as per ACSM recommendations) as being stage 1 hypertensive.

Test box: Blood pressure measurement

Position of sphygmomanometer

- Place the manometer no further than 1 m from the tester to read the scale.
- The mercury column should be vertical and at eye level.
- With the mercury manometer, errors will occur unless the eye is kept level with the top of the mercury.

Placing the cuff and stethoscope (see fig 6.2)

- Wrap the cuff around the dominant arm, so that the stethoscope will be approximately level with the heart.
- The rubber tubes from the bladder should come out of the top or the back so that the stethoscope (listening device) can be placed in the correct position just above the elbow joint at the front of the arm.
- The cuff should be 2–3 cm above where the stethoscope goes.

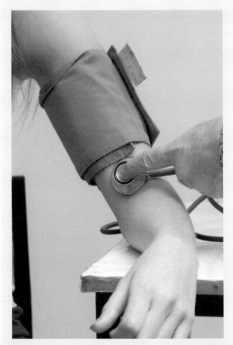

Figure 6.2 Placement of the cuff and stethoscope

Finding the starting pressure

- Find the pulse at the brachial artery.
- Inflate the cuff to a value 30 mmHg over the pressure at which the pulse disappears and immediately deflate at a rate of 2–3 mmHg per second.

- The point at which the pulse starts again is an approximation of systolic pressure. Listen out for an auscultatory gap (see table 6.2).

Auscultatory measurement of systolic and diastolic blood pressures

- Find the point of the maximum pulse at the antecubital fossa (this is where the brachial artery runs just above the elbow) and position the stethoscope.
- Hold the stethoscope firmly but without excessive pressure, as too much pressure can distort the sound.
- Inflate the cuff rapidly to about 30 mmHg above the starting level found previously, and immediately deflate at a rate of 2–3 mmHg per second.
- Sounds will now be heard, which are described in table 6.2.
- Record to the nearest 2 mmHg the level at which the first sound is heard. This should be at phase 1, which is the systolic blood pressure.
- There is now a general consensus that disappearance of sounds (phase V) should be taken as diastolic pressure.
- When all sounds have disappeared, the cuff should be deflated rapidly.

Table 6.2	Auscultatory sounds
Phase	**Description of sounds**
Phase I	The first faint, repetitive tapping sounds that gradually increase in intensity for at least two consecutive beats are the systolic blood pressure
Phase II	A brief period in which the sounds soften and acquire a swishing quality
Auscultatory gap	In some measurements, sounds may disappear for a short time
Phase III	The return of sharper sounds, which become crisper, to regain or even exceed the intensity of phase I sounds
Phase IV	The distinct, abrupt muffling of sounds, which become soft and blowing
Phase V	The point at which all sounds disappear completely is diastolic pressure

Table 6.3	Classifications of blood pressure	
	Systolic	**Diastolic**
Normal	<120 and	<80
Pre-hypertension	120–139 or	80–89
Hypertension (stage 1)	140–159 or	90–99
Hypertension (stage 2)	≥160–179 or	≥100–109

Source: Adapted from ACSM, *Guidelines for Exercise Testing and Prescription* (2009)

Table 6.4	Essential and secondary hypertension risk factors
Essential risk factor	**Comment**
Obesity	More than 85% of all individuals with hypertension have a body mass index greater than 25
High intake of dietary salt	There is a strong link between salt intake and blood pressure in that a high intake can cause blood pressure to rise
Consume a high amount of alcohol	As little as 30–40 g of alcohol per day is believed to be sufficient enough to cause hypertension
Smoking	Smoking causes vasoconstriction (blood vessels to close), which leads to hypertension
Ageing and family history	Either ageing or family history is linked to hypertension
Do not participate in regular exercise (sedentary)	Being regularly active can drastically reduce the risk of high blood pressure
Secondary risk factor	**Comment**
Cushing's syndrome	This is a condition where the adrenal glands overproduce the hormone cortisol
Coarctation of the aorta	This is a congenital defect where the artery (aorta) narrows
Conditions that cause hormone changes	These include hyperthyroidism, hypothyroidism and adrenal gland cancer
Other common causes	These include conditions such as kidney disease, obesity/metabolic disorder and pre-eclampsia (pregnancy-induced hypertension)

RISK FACTORS

For most people, there is no direct cause for their hypertension, as the condition could relate to age, ethnicity or even family history. As well as these non-modifiable risk factors, there are also several lifestyle factors that can increase the risk of developing hypertension, such as smoking and a high salt intake. Risk factors are often referred to as either essential or secondary; table 6.4 describes some of the main ones in each category.

There is an abundance of research surrounding blood pressure in relation to many other diseases, however there are common themes that are evident. For example, it is commonly agreed that, among adults aged 16 years and over, the prevalence of high blood pressure (whether it is controlled by medication or not) is affected by both increased BMI and raised waist circumference. In other words, the research agreed that overweight and obese men and women were more likely to have high blood pressure than those who were considered to be of normal weight (obese men and women being more likely than those overweight). Another common theme is that men with a raised waist circumference (more than 102 cm) have also been found to be twice as likely to have high blood pressure compared to those with a waist circumference of 102 cm or less. Women with a raised waist circumference have also been found to be more than twice as likely to have high blood pressure as those with a waist circumference of 88 cm or less.

PHYSICAL ACTIVITY BENEFITS

There is an abundance of evidence, such as that published by Kokkinos in 2000, which indicates that a programme of regular physical activity may lead to an average reduction of about 8–10 mmHg for systolic pressure and up to 7–8 mmHg for diastolic pressure. This is an important factor as, according to the *Health Survey for England* report in 2007, it has been estimated that reducing the proportion of the population with high systolic blood pressure (140 mmHg) by 50% would prevent more than 18,000 coronary heart disease events in England. In relation to the range of research in this area, even though the intensity of the physical activity that was used in many of the studies differed, depending on the level of hypertension and the fitness of the subjects, most studies used intensities below 85% of maximum heart rate (many of the studies even supported the recommendation of only going up to 80% of maximum heart rate). The age of the subjects also differed across the studies, with some showing a reduction in blood pressure even in subjects up to the age of almost 90 years. As well as the benefits of physical activity, it has also been shown in many studies that the risks associated with hypertension, such as cardiovascular events, renal disease and organ damage, can be dramatically reduced if certain lifestyle changes are implemented over a long-term period. The lifestyle changes commonly recommended include the following:

- lose weight if overweight
- reduce alcohol intake
- reduce sodium intake to less than 2.3 g per day
- maintain adequate intake of potassium, calcium and magnesium
- reduce intake of saturated fat
- stop smoking.

It should be emphasised that a multi-faceted approach that includes a regular programme of physical activity is recommended as being the optimum way in which to try to reduce the level of blood pressure of an individual. The more lifestyle approaches that are adopted, the greater the chances of success in doing so.

PHYSICAL ACTIVITY GUIDELINES

Many guidelines relating to physical activity for hypertension recommend a programme of aerobic-type activities, but resistance training is also recommended by many sources, as shown in table 6.5. It should be emphasised, though, that any physical activity recommendations should always be accompanied by advice relating to overweight, excess salt intake and alcohol consumption. For those new to physical activity, short sessions of low-intensity activity should be accumulated over the day to allow the individual to become used to the change in lifestyle. Progression should be slow and limited to 80% of maximum heart rate until the individual shows no more signs of hypertension. At the start of any physical activity session, blood pressure should be taken to check that the individual has a reading of less than 200/110 mmHg before allowing them to

Table 6.5	Physical activity guidelines for those individuals with hypertension	
	Aerobic training	**Strength training**
Mode	• Choose activities that can maximise caloric expenditure if obese	• Use an extended warm-up and gradual cool-down • Focus on muscular endurance
Intensity	• Low to moderate intensity • Up to 80%HRmax • Up to 14 RPE	• Use light loads • Overload by increasing repetitions then intensity
Duration	• 30–60 minutes per session • Increase both duration and intensity	• Perform 1 to 3 sets of 15–2RM • 1–2 minutes' rest between exercises
Frequency	• 3–7 days per week	• 2–3 sessions per week • Encourage other forms of exercise
Precautions	• Can use shorter bouts accumulated throughout the day • More than 60 minutes can diminish benefits	• Exhale on greatest effort • Avoid isometric exercises • Do not use as the only form of exercise

General precautions

- No activity should be done if resting systolic pressure is above 200 mmHg or diastolic pressure is above 110 mmHg.
- If there is a sudden drop in blood pressure during physical activity, or the individual feels dizzy or nauseous, then stop immediately.

continue. Even though it is difficult to monitor blood pressure throughout activity it is recommended that the instructor at least try if they feel that there may be a problem. The activity can always be stopped for a short period to allow for this.

BLOOD PRESSURE AND PHYSICAL ACTIVITY

Even though physical activity is recommended for hypertensive people it must be mentioned that during any form of physical exertion blood pressure can in fact increase. Blood pressure can change during both resistance training and aerobic-type activity. For example, it is generally accepted that during aerobic-type activities, systolic blood pressure increases as the work being done increases, whereas diastolic pressure usually remains about the same or in some instances can actually become lower. There is a great deal of evidence to suggest that an exaggerated blood pressure response when testing during aerobic activity may be an indication of future hypertension and even myocardial infarction. There are, however, problems associated with the measurement of blood pressure during any type of activity. For example, although systolic blood pressure can be recorded reasonably well during bicycle exercise, it is often the case that diastolic values are overestimated or underestimated. Much research has also been done on the response of blood pressure to resistance training. It has been demonstrated on many occasions that blood pressure can rise to 400/300 mmHg during maximum heavy resistance training, therefore this type of training is obviously not recommended for those with hypertension. Fig 6.3 shows typical systolic and diastolic pressure changes during aerobic activity. It can be seen in fig 6.3 that arm exercises (small muscle groups) can have a greater effect on blood pressure than larger muscle group exercises. Note also that the diastolic blood pressure is at or even below resting levels following large muscle group aerobic exercises.

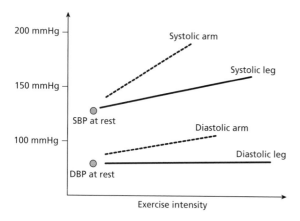

Figure 6.3 Typical systolic and diastolic pressure changes during aerobic activity

---

As blood pressure can increase during exercise it is important to stipulate that no exercise should be done if resting systolic pressure is above 200 mmHg or diastolic pressure is above 110 mmHg.

RECOMMENDED READING

American College of Sports Medicine (2009a) *ACSM's exercise management for persons with chronic diseases and disabilities* (3rd edn). Champaign, IL: Human Kinetics

American College of Sports Medicine (2009b) *ACSM's guidelines for exercise testing and prescription* (8th edn). London: Lippincott Williams & Wilkins

Beevers, G., Lip, G.Y.H. & O'Brien, E. (2001) Clinical review. ABC of hypertension. Blood pressure measurement. Part II Conventional sphygmomanometry: Technique of auscultatory blood pressure measurement. *British Medical Journal*, 322: 1043–1047

Blumenthal, J.A., Babyak, M.A., Hinderliter, A., Watkins, L.L., Craighead, L., Pao-Hwa, L., Caccia, C., Johnson, J., Waugh, R. & Sherwood, A. (2010) Effects of the DASH diet alone and in combination with exercise and weight loss on blood pressure and cardiovascular biomarkers in men and women with high blood pressure: The ENCORE study. *Archives of Internal Medicine*, 170(2): 126–135

Blumenthal, S., Epps, R.P., Heavenrich, R., Lauer, R.M., Lieberman, E., Mirkin, B., Mitchell, S.C., Boyar Naito, V., O'Hare, D., McFate Smith, W., Tarazi, R.C. & Upson, D. (1977) Report of the task force on blood pressure control in children. *Pediatrics*, 59(5): Part 2

Borg, G.A.V. (1998) *Borg's rating of perceived exertion and pain scales*. Champaign, IL: Human Kinetics

British Heart Foundation Health Promotion Research Group (2005) *Coronary heart disease statistics*. University of Oxford: Department of Public Health

Brown, B. (1993) *Heamotology, principles and procedures* (6th edn). Philadelphia, PA: Lea and Febiger

Buchalter, M. & Shapiro, L. (1991) *A colour atlas of hypertension* (2nd edn). London: Wolfe Publishing

Carretero, O.A. & Oparil, S. (2000) Essential hypertension. Part 1: Definition and etiology. *Circulation*, 101(3): 329–335

Dickson, M.E. & Sigmund, C.D. (2006) Genetic basis of hypertension: Revisiting angiotensinogen. *Hypertension*, 48(1): 14–20

Ehrman, J.K., Gordon, P.M., Visich, P.S. & Keteyian, S.J. (2003) *Clinical exercise physiology*. Champaign, IL: Human Kinetics

Elliott, W.J. (2003) The economic impact of hypertension. *Journal of Clinical Hypertension*, 5(4): 3–13

Health Survey for England (2007) *Healthy lifestyles: Knowledge, attitudes and behaviour.* Leeds: NHS Information Centre for Health and Social Care

Joint British Societies (2005) Guidelines on prevention of cardiovascular disease in clinical practice. *Heart*, 91(V)

Joint Health Surveys Unit (2004) *The Health Survey for England 2003.* Royal Free and University College Medical School: Department of Health

Kearney, P.M., Whelton, M., Reynolds, K., Muntner, P., Whelton, P.K. & He, J. (2005) Global burden of hypertension: Analysis of worldwide data. *Lancet*, 365(9455): 217–223

Kokkinos, P.F. (2000) Exercise as hypertension therapy. *Hellenic Journal of Cardiology*, 42: 182–192

Lackland, D.T. & Egan, B.M. (2007) Dietary salt restriction and blood pressure in clinical trials. *Current Hypertension Reports*, 9(4): 314–319

NHS Information Centre, Lifestyle Statistics (2009) *Statistics on obesity, physical activity and diet: England, February 2009.* London: NHS Information Centre for Health and Social Care

Papadakis, M.A., McPhee, S.J. & Tierney, L.M. (2008) *Current medical diagnosis and treatment.* New York: McGraw-Hill

Rahmouni, K., Correia, M.L., Haynes, W.G. & Mark, A.L. (2005) Obesity-associated hypertension: New insights into mechanisms. *Hypertension*, 45(1): 9–14

Rosengren, A., Hawken, S., Ounpuu, S., Sliwa, K., Zubaid, M., Almahmeed, W.A., Blackett, K.N., Sitthi-amorn, C., Sato, H. & Yusuf, S. (2004) Association of psychosocial risk factors with risk of acute myocardial infarction in 11119 cases and 13648 controls from 52 countries (the INTERHEART study): Case-control study. *Lancet*, 364: 953–962

Sagnella, G.A. & Swift, P.A. (2006) The renal epithelial sodium channel: Genetic heterogeneity and implications for the treatment of high blood pressure. *Current Pharmaceutical Design*, 12(14): 2221–2234

Segura, J. & Ruilope, L.M. (2007) Obesity, essential hypertension and renin-angiotensin system. *Public Health Nutrition*, 10(10A): 1151–1155

Shankie, S. (2001) *Hypertension in focus.* Pharmaceutical Press. London: Stationery Office

Solomon, E.P., Schmidt, R.R. & Adragna, P.J. (1990) *Human anatomy and physiology* (2nd edn). Philadelphia, PA: Saunders College Publishing

Thibodeau, G. & Patton, K. (2003) *Anatomy and physiology* (5th edn). St Louis: Mosby, Inc.

Torrata, G. & Derrickson, B. (2009) *Principles of anatomy and physiology* (12th edn). New Jersey: John Wiley & Sons

Wilmore, J.H. & Costill, D.L. (2005) *Physiology of sport and exercise* (3rd edn). Champaign, IL: Human Kinetics

Yusuf, S., Hawken, S., Ounpuu, S., Dans, T., Avezum, A., Lanas, F., McQueen, M., Budaj, A., Pais, P., Varigos, J. & Lisheng, L. (2004) Effect of potentially modifiable risk factors associated with myocardial infarction in 52 countries (the INTERHEART study): Case-control study. *Lancet*, 364: 937–952

USEFUL WEBSITES

American College of Sports Medicine – www.acsm.org
British Heart Foundation – www.bhf.org.uk
British Hypertension Society – www.bhsoc.org
Department of Health – www.dh.gov.uk
European Society of Hypertension – www.eshonline.org
NHS Information Centre – www.ic.nhs.uk

HYPERLIPIDAEMIA

7

KEYPOINTS

- The general term 'hyperlipidaemia' refers to increased levels of lipids in the blood.
- Lipids come in various forms, such as triglycerides or different types of cholesterol.
- Hyperlipidaemia can be classified into two subcategories (hypertriglyceridaemia or hypercholesterolaemia), depending on whether triglyceride levels or cholesterol levels are high.
- Over 60% of CHD and around 40% of ischemic stroke in developed countries are due to total blood cholesterol levels in excess of 3.8 mmol/l.
- It is estimated that 45% of heart attacks in western Europe and 35% of heart attacks in central and eastern Europe are due to abnormal blood lipids.
- Those with abnormal lipids have a threefold higher risk of a heart attack compared to those with normal lipids.
- Average total blood cholesterol level for men aged 16 and above in England is generally thought to be about 5.5 mmol/l and for women 5.6 mmol/l, however about 66% of men and women have blood cholesterol levels of 5.0 mmol/l and above.
- The average HDL-cholesterol level for men aged 16 and above in England is about 1.4 mmol/l and 1.6 mmol/l for women. Overall, about 17% of men and 2% of women have HDL-cholesterol levels of less than 1.0 mmol/l; GPs generally recommend treatment for those with concentrations below this level.
- Levels of less than 1.0 mmol/l for men in other countries range from 7 to 9% in France, about 15% in Germany, 15–23% in Holland, 24% in India, 30% in Canada, 7–38% in the USA and 75% in Thailand.
- It has been shown that regular participation in exercise can have many beneficial effects, including the following:
  - reduction in triglyceride concentrations
  - increase in HDL-cholesterol concentrations
  - increase in enzyme activity for metabolisation of lipoprotein.

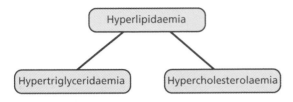

Figure 7.1 Classifications of hyperlipidaemia

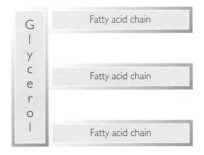

Figure 7.2 A typical triglyceride

WHAT IS IT?

The general term 'hyperlipidaemia' is taken from the Greek word 'hyper' meaning more than and 'lipid' meaning fat, and refers to increased levels of lipids in the blood. Lipids come in various forms such as triglycerides or different types of cholesterol. As can be seen in fig 7.1, hyperlipidaemia can be classified into two subcategories (hypertriglyceridaemia or hypercholesterolaemia) depending on whether triglyceride levels or cholesterol levels are high.

TRIGLYCERIDE

This is a type of lipid that is derived from fats in certain foods such as meat products but can also be made in the body from other food sources like carbohydrates. All food can be broken down in the body to provide energy, but if too much food is eaten and is not used immediately for energy, it can be broken down into fatty acids and transported to fat cells, where it is converted to triglyceride to be stored for future energy use. As can be seen in fig 7.2, triglycerides are made up of a substance called glycerol and three fatty acid chains. It is the make-up of the fatty acid chains that determines if the triglyceride is a 'saturated' or 'unsaturated' type, which are two main classifications of fats.

CHOLESTEROL

This is a type of lipid found in all of us, as it is an essential compound needed for important roles in the body such as making cells (the body's 'building blocks') and hormones (which act as important chemical messengers in the body). Both triglycerides and cholesterol move between the intestine and the liver via the bloodstream. On their own they are not soluble in the blood, therefore they must combine with protein to form various lipoproteins in order to be transported through the blood. When blood is being tested for cholesterol levels it is really the lipoproteins that are being measured. The main types of lipoproteins that are often measured are known as:

- very low-density lipoprotein (VLDL), which is the main carrier of triglyceride;
- low-density lipoprotein (LDL), which is the 'bad' carrier of cholesterol and
- high-density lipoprotein (HDL), known as the 'good' carrier of cholesterol.

High lipid levels in the blood are known to speed up a process called 'atherosclerosis', or hardening of the arteries. Arteries, if undamaged, are normally smooth on the inside, which allows blood to flow easily through them. If the arteries get damaged in any way (smoking can cause damage, for example), a substance called 'plaque' can form on the inside walls at the site of the damage. Plaque is just the collective term for substances such as lipids that can 'stick' to the artery walls as they flow through the bloodstream. If plaque continues to build up (as can be seen in fig 7.3), the arteries can narrow and stiffen, which in turn can reduce the blood flow and lead to serious consequences such as stroke and heart attack.

An abundance of research has been done relating to the effects of cholesterol and plaque build-up. Much evidence shows that it is excess levels of the 'bad' LDL-cholesterol that is linked to deposits on the arteries, whereas it is thought that 'good' HDL-cholesterol carries any excess cholesterol away from the arteries and back to the liver, where it is broken down and recycled. As a result of the research, therefore, having a high level of HDL-cholesterol is considered to be a good thing. High levels of cholesterol in the blood can be caused by a range of different factors. For example, in some people, a high cholesterol concentration is caused by an inherited genetic defect. If this is the case, it is known as familial hypercholesterolaemia (FH) and makes up about 60% of all known hyperlipidaemia cases. The other 40% of cases are known as secondary hyperlipidaemia. This particular category is usually linked to some kind of metabolic disease, such as diabetes, or can result from certain dietary factors such as a high intake of fat or carbohydrate in the diet, or even as a result of alcohol abuse.

PREVALENCE

Even though the estimated numbers of people with abnormal lipid levels varies according to the source, recognised health bodies such as the British Heart Foundation (BHF) and the World Health Organization (WHO) agree that the risk of coronary heart disease (CHD) is directly related to blood cholesterol levels. Other reports, such as *The World Health Report* in 2002, have estimated that around 8% of all the disease burden in developed countries was caused by raised blood cholesterol. This report also stated that over 60% of CHD and around 40% of ischaemic stroke (see chapter 13) in developed countries was due to total blood cholesterol levels being in excess of 3.8 mmol/l (see table 7.2 on page 98 for the classification of cholesterol levels). More recently, in the 2004 INTERHEART case-control study, it was estimated that 45% of heart attacks in western Europe and 35% of heart attacks in central and eastern Europe were due to abnormal blood lipid levels, and that those with abnormal lipid levels had a threefold higher risk of a heart attack compared to those with normal lipid levels. According to the *Health Survey for England* in 2003 the average total blood cholesterol level for men aged 16 years and above (in England) was generally thought to be about 5.5 mmol/l and for women it was 5.6 mmol/l, however about 66% of men and women had blood cholesterol levels of

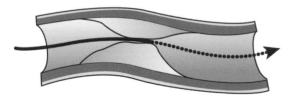

Figure 7.3 An artery wall with plaque build-up

5.0 mmol/l and above. The survey also stated that the average HDL-cholesterol level for men aged 16 years and above in England was about 1.4 mmol/l and for women about 1.6 mmol/l. Interestingly, it was reported that, overall, about 17% of men and 2% of women had HDL-cholesterol levels of less than 1.0 mmol/l. Those below this level are generally recommended for treatment. Comparisons can be made to the numbers of men in other countries with levels of less than 1.0 mmol/l. For example, this ranges between 7 and 9% in France, about 15% in Germany, 15 to 23% in Holland, 24% in India, 30% in Canada, 7 to 38% in the USA and 75% in Thailand.

SYMPTOMS

This particular condition has no noticeably obvious symptoms and is normally found only during a routine blood test or if the person has suffered some other condition such as a stroke or heart attack. Having said that, deposits of cholesterol (known as xanthomas) can form, although the occurrence is seldom, under the skin (around the eyes or in the Achilles tendon) in those people who have very high levels of blood cholesterol.

DIAGNOSIS

A clinical diagnosis of hypercholesterolaemia is typically based on a combination of methods such as a medical history screening, a physical examination and blood tests that are carried out with certain conditions (normally overnight

fasting). Initially, if a random blood test indicates a total cholesterol level that is high, a further test is normally done that is more specific. This more specific blood test is done in order to determine the individual levels of LDL-cholesterol, HDL-cholesterol and triglycerides as the ratio between them is important. For example, if a person with a borderline high total cholesterol level has a good ratio of LDL to HDL then it is considered to be healthier than having a borderline high total cholesterol level with a poor ratio of LDL to HDL. It is also useful to know the individual levels of HDL-cholesterol, LDL-cholesterol and triglycerides, as various lifestyle factors and medication have different effects on them, which will inform the GP as to the appropriate course of action. Once blood tests have been carried out, the GP will normally use a classification table (such as tables 7.1 and 7.2) to determine the risk level of the individual. It should be noted, however, that classifications will vary depending on the publication source.

Even though the classification levels in tables 7.1 and 7.2 are a typical representation of many published guidelines, according to the Joint British Societies (JBS) in 2005, the optimal total cholesterol target for the population should be 4.0 mmol/l and LDL cholesterol target should be 2.0 mmol/l, or a 25% reduction in total cholesterol and a 30% reduction in LDL-cholesterol (whichever gets the person to the lowest absolute value). These targets were published following an amalgamation of several bodies to form the JBS. They were the British Cardiac Society, the British Hypertension Society, HEART UK, Diabetes UK, the Primary Care Cardiovascular Society and the Stroke Association. The main role of the JBS following the amalgamation is to provide expert

Test box: Blood lipids

Equipment needed

There are various types of blood lipid testing kits available, such as the Roche Reflotron®. Once blood has been analysed, compare the triglyceride levels to the classifications in table 7.1.

Table 7.1	Triglyceride classification (units are mmol/l of blood)
Classification	**Levels**
Normal	<1.69 mmol/l
Borderline high	1.69 to 2.25 mmol/l
High	2.26 to 5.63 mmol/l
Very high	>5.63 mmol/l

Once blood has been analysed, compare the cholesterol levels to the classifications in table 7.2.

Table 7.2	Cholesterol classifications (units are mmol/l of blood)		
Lipoprotein	**Desirable**	**Border**	**Abnormal**
Total cholesterol	<5.2	5.2–6.5	>6.5
LDL-cholesterol	<3.0	3.0–5.0	>5.0
HDL-cholesterol	>1.0	0.9–1.0	<0.9

advice in relation to all aspects of cardiovascular disease and, in particular, strategies for the prevention of the disease.

RISK FACTORS

It is generally accepted that there is a genetic link to the development of hyperlipidaemia, but there are many other factors that can contribute to the development, albeit in varying degrees. E.g. it has been suggested that gene mutations (which are a genetic link) can result in either an overproduction or defective clearance of triglyceride and LDL-cholesterol, or in underproduction or excessive clearance of HDL-cholesterol. In other words, ultimately resulting in high levels of LDL-cholesterol (baddies) and low levels of HDL-cholesterol (goodies). In the case of those with familial hypercholesterolaemia (FH), as described earlier, raised blood cholesterol levels are present from birth, and may lead to early development of atherosclerosis and coronary heart disease. Some statistics show that siblings and children of a person with FH can have as much as a 50% risk of inheriting the condition. Apart from the genetic link, some of the main risk factors include a sedentary lifestyle, an excessive dietary intake of saturated fat, cholesterol and trans fats (these are fats that are commonly used in many processed foods), or high intake of carbohydrates. There are many other common risk factors, which include smoking, hypertension, diabetes mellitus, alcohol overuse, chronic kidney disease, hypothyroidism, primary biliary cirrhosis and other cholestatic liver diseases. There is also a wide range of certain drugs, such as thiazides, beta-blockers, retinoids, highly active antiretroviral agents, oestrogen and progestins, and glucocorticoids, which can also increase the risk of development of the condition.

PHYSICAL ACTIVITY BENEFITS

Research in this particular area is abundant. Generally it has been shown that regular participation in physical activity can have many beneficial effects, including the following:

- a reduction in triglyceride concentrations
- an increase in HDL-cholesterol concentrations
- an increase in enzyme activity for metabolisation of lipoprotein (a better ability to break down and use).

In particular, investigations, such as those by Shern-Brewer *et al.* (1998), Tomas *et al.* (2002) and Vasankari *et al.* (2000), have shown a reduction in LDL-cholesterol levels in individuals as a result of them participating in a regular programme of physical activity. It is important to

remember, however, that there may be substantially different responses to physical activity regimes in individuals with congenital deficiencies in lipid transport. It is also important to be aware that there is a range of lipid-lowering prescribed medications such as fibric acid derivatives that, when used in conjunction with a programme of physical activity, can increase the risk of muscle damage. Other research shows that the adverse effect of other drugs such as beta blockers may be reduced by physical activity. It is prudent, therefore, to seek medical advice regarding the use of medication for the treatment of hyperlipidaemia in conjunction with any form of physical activity.

PHYSICAL ACTIVITY GUIDELINES

Those with hyperlipidaemia should combine physical activity with a lifestyle that restricts energy intake and dietary fat consumption. Although there is a great deal of variation between individuals with regard to the effects of physical activity on blood lipids, most people can expect a favourable change within several months of starting a programme. Intensity should be kept low to start with and progression should be generally slow depending on the individual. Adherence to activity is essential for this population as single one-off sessions have little impact in the long term (see table 7.3, overleaf).

Table 7.3	Physical activity guidelines for those with hyperlipidaemia	
	Aerobic training	**Strength training**
Mode	• Choose activities that can maximise caloric expenditure if obese, and weight bearing if not	• Use an extended warm-up and gradual cool-down • Focus on muscular endurance
Intensity	• Low to moderate intensity • 50–80%HRmax • 8–14 RPE	• Use light loads • Overload by increasing repetitions then intensity
Duration	• Up to 40 minutes per session • Increase intensity with slow progression	• Perform 1 to 3 sets of 15–20 RM • 1–2 minutes' rest between exercises
Frequency	• 5 days per week	• 2–3 sessions per week • Encourage other forms of exercise
Precautions	• May need to use perceived exertion for monitoring intensity • Intensity seems to have less of an effect than the total amount of kcals spent doing the activity	• Resistance exercise training alone does positively influence blood lipid levels, but not as significantly as cardiovascular activity

General precautions

• Blood lipid changes after one activity session do not last long and are lost within **48** hours, therefore regular activity needs to be maintained.

• Generally, fitter people need to do activities more often to influence lipid levels.

• About 300 to 500 kcals spent in a single session may be enough to improve blood lipid levels of less fit people, whereas 800 to 1000 kcals may be required for those who are fitter.

• When weight loss and physical activity are combined, they can have an additive effect on reducing LDL and triglyceride levels, and increasing HDL.

• Aerobic activity for managing blood lipid levels should be designed to produce a caloric expenditure of 1200 to 2000 kcals per week.

RECOMMENDED READING

American College of Sports Medicine (2009a) *ACSM's exercise management for persons with chronic diseases and disabilities* (3rd edn). Champaign, IL: Human Kinetics

American College of Sports Medicine (2009b) *ACSM's guidelines for exercise testing and prescription* (8th edn). London: Lippincott Williams & Wilkins

British Heart Foundation Health Promotion Research Group (2005) *Coronary heart disease statistics*. University of Oxford: Department of Public Health

Durrington, P. (2003) Dyslipidaemia. *Lancet*, 362(9385): 717–731

Gami, A. (2006) Secondary prevention of ischaemic cardiac events. *Clinical Evidence*, 15: 195–228

Grundy, S.M., Balady, G.J., Criqui, M.H., Fletcher, G., Greenland, P., Hiratzka, L.F., Houston-Miller, N.,

Kris-Etherton, P., Krumholz, H.M., LaRosa, J., Ockene, I.S., Pearson, T.A., Reed, J. & Washington, R. (1998) Primary prevention of coronary heart disease: Guidance from Framingham: A statement for healthcare professionals from the AHA Task Force on Risk Reduction. American Heart Association. *Circulation*, 97(18): 1876–1887

Hayward, R.A., Hofer, T.P. & Vijan, S. (2006) Narrative review: Lack of evidence for recommended low-density lipoprotein treatment targets: A solvable problem. *Annals of Internal Medicine*, 145(7): 520–530

Joint British Societies (2005) Guidelines on prevention of cardiovascular disease in clinical practice. *Heart*, 91(V)

Joint Health Surveys Unit (2004) *The Health Survey for England 2003*. Royal Free and University College Medical School: Department of Health

Kausik, K.R., Seshasai, S.R.K., Erqou, S., Sever, P., Jukema, W., Ford, I. & Sattar, N. (2010) Statins and all-cause mortality in high-risk primary prevention: A meta-analysis of 11 randomized controlled trials involving 65 229 participants. *Archives of Internal Medicine*, 170(12): 1024

McMurry, M.P., Cerqueira, M.T., Connor, S.L. & Connor, W.E. (1991) Changes in lipid and lipoprotein levels and body weight in Tarahumara Indians after consumption of an affluent diet. *New England Journal of Medicine*, 325(24): 1704–1708

Mozaffarian, D., Katan, M.B., Ascherio, A., Stampfer, M.J. & Willett, W.C. (2006) Trans-fatty acids and cardiovascular disease. *New England Journal of Medicine*, 354(15): 1601–1613

National Institute for Health and Clinical Excellence (NICE) (2010) *Lipid modification: Cardiovascular risk assessment and the modification of blood lipids for the primary and secondary prevention of cardiovascular disease.* NICE Clinical Guideline 67. London: NICE

Pignone, M. (2005) Primary prevention: Dyslipidaemia. *Clinical Evidence*, 14: 142–150

Pignone, M., Phillips, C., Atkins, D., Teutsch, S., Mulrow, C. & Lohr, K. (2001) Screening and treating adults for lipid disorders. *American Journal of Preventative Medicine*, 20(3, suppl.): 77–89

Shern-Brewer, R., Santanam, N., Wetzstein, C., White-Welkley, J. & Parthasarathy, S. (1998) Exercise and cardiovascular disease: A new perspective. *Arteriosclerosis Thrombosis and Vascular Biology*, 18: 1181–1187

Snow, V., Aronson, M., Hornbake, E., Mottur-Pilson, C. & Weiss, K. (2004) Lipid control in the management of type 2 diabetes mellitus: A clinical practice guideline from the American College of Physicians. *Annals of Internal Medicine*, 140(8): 644–649

Starc, T.J., Shea, S., Cohn, L.C., Mosca, L., Gersony, W.M. & Deckelbaum, R.J. (1998) Greater dietary intake of simple carbohydrate is associated with lower concentrations of high-density-lipoprotein cholesterol in hypercholesterolemic children. *American Journal of Clinical Nutrition*, 67: 1147–1154

Tang, J.L., Armitage, J.M., Lancaster, T., Silagy, C.A., Fowler, G.H. & Neil, H.A. (1998) Systematic review of dietary intervention trials to lower blood total cholesterol in free-living subjects. *British Medical Journal*, 316(7139): 1213–1220

Tomas, M., Elosua, R., Senti, M., Vila, J., Anglada, R., Fitó, M., Covas, M.I. & Marrugat, J. (2002) Paraoxonase1–192 polymorphism modulates the effects of regular and acute exercise on paraoxonase1 activity. *Journal of Lipid Research*, 43(5): 7137–7120

Vasankari, T., Lehtonen-Veromaa, M., Mottonen, T., Ahotupa, M., Irjala, K., Heinonen, O., Leino, A. & Viikari, J. (2000) Reduced mildly oxidized LDL in young female athletes. *Atherosclerosis*, 151: 399–405

Vijan, S. & Hayward, R.A. (2004) Pharmacologic lipid-lowering therapy in type 2 diabetes mellitus: Background paper for the American College of Physicians. *Annals of Internal Medicine*, 140(8): 650–658

Weingärtner, O., Bohm, M. & Laufs, U. (2009) Controversial role of plant sterol esters in the management of hypercholesterolaemia. *European Heart Journal*, 30(4): 404–409

Yusuf, S., Hawken, S., Ounpuu, S., Dans, T., Avezum, A., Lanas, F., McQueen, M., Budaj, A., Pais, P., Varigos, J. & Lisheng, L. (2004) Effect of potentially modifiable risk factors associated with myocardial infarction in 52 countries (the INTERHEART study): Case-control study. *Lancet*, 364: 937–952

USEFUL WEBSITES

American Heart Association – www.americanheart.org
British Heart Foundation – www.bhf.org.uk
Department of Health – www.dh.gov.uk
Food Standards Agency – www.food.gov.uk
National Health Service – www.nhs.uk
National Institute for Health and Clinical Excellence –
    www.nice.org

ARTHRITIS

8

KEYPOINTS

- Arthritis (in all forms) affects about 7 million people in the UK.
- Osteoarthritis is more common in men before the age of 45 years and more common in women after the age of 45 years.
- Rheumatoid arthritis is thought to affect about 2–3% of the UK population.
- Gout is thought to affect around 1% of the western population at some point in their lives (usually age 20 and older) and has increased in frequency in recent decades.
- Men are affected by ankylosing spondylitis more than women, by a ratio of about three to one.
- The occurrence of lupus in northern Europe is about 40 in every 100,000, and affects females more than men by a ratio of about nine to one.
- Men between the ages of 40 and 50 years are more likely to develop gout than women, who rarely develop the disorder before the age of menopause.
- There is little evidence to show that physical activity can prevent osteoarthritis.
- Both absence of and an excess of stress on the joints can increase the risk of osteoarthritis.
- Physical activity can have beneficial effects for people with osteoarthritis, including those who have had a joint replacement, but too much physical activity can be detrimental.
- As a general rule, when any form of arthritis is at its most painful (i.e. flares up) physical activity levels should be low.

WHAT IS IT?

Arthritis is an extremely common disease that generally relates to the swelling or inflammation of a joint. The term comes from the Greek 'arth' meaning joint and 'itis' meaning inflammation. There are over 200 forms (known as rheumatological diseases) of which the two most common are osteoarthritis, which is classed as a degenerative joint disease, and rheumatoid arthritis, which is a multi-joint inflammatory disease.

OSTEOARTHRITIS

This particular form of arthritis is localised or specific to a particular joint (for example, the knee joint or the hip joint). Over a long period of time, 'wear and tear' can affect the articular cartilage that covers the ends of bones that come together at a joint. Articular cartilage is normally smooth and hard so that the bones in a joint can slide across each other without too much friction. Unfortunately, though, the cartilage is not very thick and is not designed to withstand many years of repetitive movement, especially if done with any form of impact, as this can cause the cartilage to wear away and eventually leave the bone

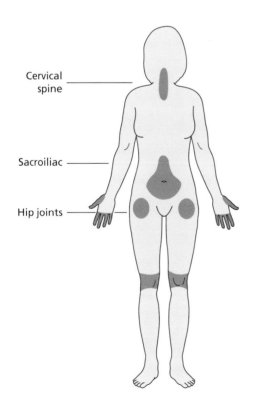

Cervical spine

Sacroiliac

Hip joints

Figure 8.1 Common sites of osteoarthritis

underneath exposed. When cartilage does wear away, bony spurs and growths (known as osteophytes) can develop, which can break off and float around inside the joint space. Not only does this cause pain with any movement, but inflammation and swelling can occur around the joint as a response mechanism in order to protect it. Fig 8.1 shows typical joints in the body that are commonly affected by osteoarthritis.

RHEUMATOID ARTHRITIS

The other main form of arthritis is known as 'rheumatoid arthritis' and is classed as an inflammatory disease that may affect several joints and other organ systems in the body. It is thought that this occurs as a result of the immune system attacking the body's own tissues. The reasons for this are not fully understood, but it is thought to either have some kind of genetic link or can otherwise be caused by a viral or bacterial infection. Rheumatoid arthritis can affect any joint in the body, but the joints commonly affected are the fingers, knees, wrists and elbows. The disease is generally more common in women than it is in men, and even though it can occur in younger age people, it is more prevalent in older age. The pain associated with this disease can be quite severe, especially in the morning. Pain is felt as a result of the wearing away (erosion) of bone and cartilage around the affected joint leading to inflammation and swelling, as it is with osteoarthritis. A comparison between a typical joint and an affected joint can be seen in fig 8.2 overleaf.

As well as the two main types of arthritis, there are several other less common forms of the disease. It is possible that those supervising physical activity may have to deal with individuals who have one of the other forms. It is recommended,

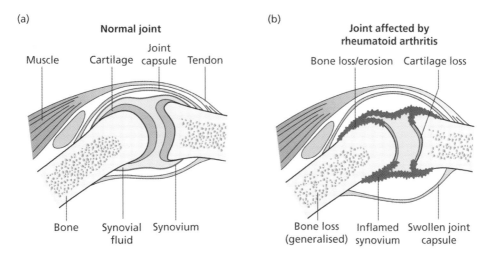

(a) **Normal joint**

Muscle Cartilage Joint capsule Tendon

Bone Synovial fluid Synovium

(b) **Joint affected by rheumatoid arthritis**

Bone loss/erosion Cartilage loss

Bone loss (generalised) Inflamed synovium Swollen joint capsule

Figure 8.2 A normal joint and a joint affected by rheumatoid arthritis

therefore, that even if there is less chance of supervising someone with another form of arthritis, a degree of familiarity is still needed on the part of the supervisor. Some of the other more common forms of arthritis include lupus, gout and ankylosing spondylitis.

LUPUS

The correct term for this particular disease is 'lupus erythematosus', which is actually the term given to a collection of diseases in which there are underlying problems with the immune system. A disease such as this is more generally known in collective terms as an 'autoimmune disease'. Some forms of lupus can affect many different body systems other than joints. Systems such as the skin, kidneys, blood cells, heart and lungs can be affected. Currently there is no known cure for the disease and those with it can go through periods of illness (known as flares) and periods of remission (when there are no symptoms). As with rheumatoid arthritis, those people with lupus suffer from inflammation of the joints, in particular the hands, knees, elbows and feet.

GOUT

It is commonly understood that the form of arthritis known as 'gout' is caused when high levels of uric acid (which is a waste product) in the blood are crystallised and deposited in a joint, causing inflammation, and in the long term it can lead to bone erosion. A high level of uric acid in the blood is known as 'hyperuricaemia' and in the early stages of gout it usually occurs only in one joint, but with time can occur in many joints and be quite severe. The joints that are affected by gout can often become swollen as chalky deposits of uric acid (known as 'tophi') can result in lumps under the skin. These lumps can then cause the joint to lose function and range of movement. Kidney stones are also a common problem with this disease as it is the kidneys that filter the high levels of uric acid. The joint at the base of the big toe (the metatarsal-phalangeal joint) is the most commonly affected in those people with gout as this occurs in around half of all cases of gout. When gout affects the big toe it is known as 'podagra'.

ANKYLOSING SPONDYLITIS

The term 'ankylosing spondylitis' comes from the Greek 'ankylos' meaning bent and 'spondylos' meaning vertebrae. It is a disease that is classed as a chronic, inflammatory arthritis and autoimmune disease. Ankylosing spondylitis mainly affects joints in the spine and at the sacroilium (joint between the spine and pelvis). The long-term effects of this disease are quite severe as they can result in fusion of the spine (this is where some of the vertebrae in the spine are fused or joined together). A complete fusion of the spine is commonly known as 'bamboo spine'. Men are affected by this disease more than women, by a ratio of about of three to one. Related symptoms typically start to appear between the age of about 20 and 40 years. The main symptoms of ankylosing

spondylitis include chronic pain and stiffness in the lower part of the spine, which can sometimes affect the entire spine and sacroilium. It is a common occurrence that pain is referred to one or other buttock or the back of the thigh. In about 40% of cases, symptoms include inflammation of the eye, which can cause redness and loss of vision. Table 8.1 gives a summary and brief description of the common forms of arthritis.

PREVALENCE

It is difficult to estimate the numbers of people with arthritis as not all of those with the disease seek any medical help or advice. However, according to the Arthritis Research Campaign in 2002, arthritis (in all forms) affects about 7 million people (which is more than 10%) in the UK at any one time. The National Institute of Arthritis and Musculoskeletal and Skin Diseases reported in 2002 that osteoarthritis was more common in

Table 8.1	Overview of common types of arthritis		
Disease	**Disease type**	**Commonly affected joints**	**Relation to physical activity**
Osteoarthritis	Local degeneration	Hands, spine, hips, knees	Joint pain, stiffness, cartilage erosion
Rheumatoid arthritis	Inflammatory	Wrist, hands, knees, feet, neck	Morning stiffness, inflammation, joint instability
Lupus	Inflammatory	Hands, knees, elbows, feet	Arthralgia, fatigue
Gout	Crystal deposits	Big toe, ankles, knees, wrists	Joint inflammation, pain
Ankylosing spondylitis	Inflammatory	Spine, hip, shoulder girdle, knees	Pain, spinal fusion

Source: Adapted from ACSM (2009)

men before the age of 45 years and more common in women after the age of 45 years. The report also stated that, for those with osteoarthritis, the ratio of young (16–44 years), middle aged (45–64 years) and older age (65+ years) people that had the disease in the UK was reported to be 1:6:9 respectively, which shows that the disease is more prevalent in older age. Rheumatoid arthritis is thought to affect about 2–3% of the UK population, whereas gout is thought to affect around 1% of the entire western population at some point in their lives (usually at age 20 and older) and has increased in frequency in recent decades. Men, particularly those between the ages of 40 and 50 years, are more likely to develop gout than women, who rarely develop the disorder before the age of menopause. In the case of lupus, the rate in northern Europe is about 40 in every 100,000, and it affects females more than men at a rate of about nine to one.

SYMPTOMS

Irrespective of the type of arthritis an individual has, the common symptoms for all arthritis disorders include those shown in table 8.2. It can also be seen that those disorders such as lupus, rheumatoid arthritis and gout can affect other organs in the body, leading to a variety of different symptoms other than the common ones described.

It can be seen in table 8.2 that most of the forms of arthritis relate to some sort of joint swelling or inflammation as being symptomatic of the disease. The degree of severity of the inflammation is, however, very different among individuals as it can range from mild inflammation that doesn't cause much movement restriction or pain to very severe inflammation that can dramatically reduce function and range of movement and cause a great deal of pain. Fig 8.3 shows a typical example of swelling in the joints of the fingers due to rheumatoid arthritis, which can reduce both the function (strength, dexterity, etc.) and range of movement.

Table 8.2	Common and specific symptoms of arthritis	
Common arthritis symptoms	**Lupus and rheumatoid arthritis symptoms**	**Gout symptoms**
• Varied levels of pain	• Lack of dexterity or walking problems	• Hyperuricaemia (high levels of uric acid in the blood)
• Swelling and deformity	• Fatigue	• Uric acid crystals in the joint fluid
• Joint stiffness	• Unexplained fever	
• Constant joint ache	• Weight loss	• Repeat attacks of acute arthritis
• Muscle weakness	• Poor sleep	• Arthritis that develops in a day, producing a swollen, warm joint
• Loss of flexibility	• Muscle aches and pains	
• Decreased aerobic fitness (as a consequence)	• Tenderness and swollen joints and glands	• Attack of arthritis in only one joint in the early stages (mainly toe, ankle or knee)
	• Hair loss	
	• Red rashes	

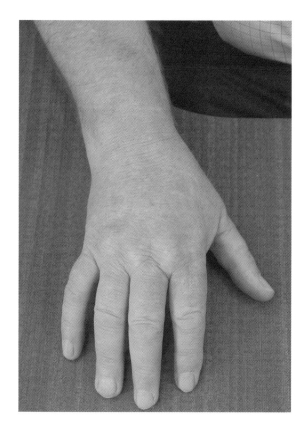

Figure 8.3 Example of swelling due to rheumatoid arthritis

RISK FACTORS

As many of the forms of arthritis relate to immune system problems with no particular cause, it is difficult to identify any risk factors that can be modified. In other words, it is difficult to find something that can be done to reduce the risk potential. Research, therefore, as well as investigating the immune dysfunction problems, has also focused on the few potentially modifiable risk factors that are associated with particular arthritis forms.

RISK OF OSTEOARTHRITIS

In the case of osteoarthritis, however, the disease is not related to an immune system problem, therefore there are several risk factors that have been identified as being thought to be modifiable to a certain extent in order to reduce the risk potential. The main risk factors that have been identified are the following:

- prior joint trauma (injuries)
- obesity
- repetitive joint use
- sedentary lifestyle
- ageing
- regular high-intensity activity levels
- regular high-impact activities.

It is generally thought that there is no excess risk of osteoarthritis in individuals who participate in regular moderate-intensity activities such as walking, cycling and swimming, and indeed the risk may even be lowered. However, increased risk is associated with higher levels of regular physical activities such as track and field athletics and a variety of sports. In order to distinguish between what are considered to be moderate and higher levels of physical activity, the Department of Health stated in 2004 that there appears to be an activity threshold level above which the risk of osteoarthritis is particularly high. This was suggested to be either 3 hours of heavy physical activity per day, or at least 20 miles of weekly running (for knee and hip osteoarthritis). This is slightly different to the investigation by Lueponsak and colleagues in 2002, who suggested that there is an increased risk of hip and knee osteoarthritis once people cross a particular threshold, which could be as low as 10 flights of stairs per day. Also, it is not just a higher threshold level that seems to exist, as research by Pope *et al.* in 2003 found that both the absence of and an excess of stress on the joints can influence the risk of osteoarthritis.

RISK OF RHEUMATOID ARTHRITIS

This particular disease is related to the immune system, therefore physical activity does not have an effect on the potential risk. Women are generally considered to be two to three times more likely to develop the disease than men, especially between the ages of 40 and 60 years. A family history of the disease is also thought to increase the risk. For example, it is thought that siblings of those with the disease are five to ten times more susceptible. Scientists suggest that the disease is not inherited directly as it is more likely to be a predisposition to the disease that is inherited. Smoking is considered another risk factor for rheumatoid arthritis even though the exact mechanism of this is not fully understood.

RISK OF GOUT

In the case of reducing the risk of gout, diet plays an important part for everyone. Being overweight is one of the main risk factors for developing the disease as it has been found that excess fat in the body can lead to an overproduction of uric acid. In terms of the types of food we eat, eating foods rich in 'purines' can lead to more problems with the disease. A purine is just the name given to certain compounds containing nitrogen that occur naturally in food. The reason for this is that purines are broken down into uric acid, which is the substance that is potentially responsible for gout. Purines can be found in both meat and non-meat sources, as shown in table 8.3. It is

Table 8.3	Foods rich in purines
Non-meat sources	**Meat and fish sources**
Anchovies	Beef kidneys
Asparagus	Brains
Dried beans and	Game meats
peas	Herring
Gravy	Liver
Mushrooms	Mackerel/sardines
Sweetbreads	Scallops

sensible advice, therefore, not to have a regular diet that is high in purine-rich foods as this could substantially increase the risk of developing the disease, or exacerbate the disease in those people who already have gout. Drinking heavily (alcohol) has also been identified as a modifiable risk factor as it can negatively affect the removal of uric acid from the body. Both one-off 'binges' and long-term abuse should be discouraged, not just from the perspective of risk of gout but for many other health reasons as well. Research shows that having high blood pressure has also been linked to an increased risk of developing the disease. Even though there are several modifiable risk factors associated with gout (eating, drinking, high blood pressure, overweight, etc.), genetics has been found to play a fairly major role, as about 20% of those that have been diagnosed have displayed a degree of family history of the disease.

RISK OF LUPUS

There are several potential risk factors that can affect an individual's chance of developing lupus, such as those listed in table 8.4. Most of the risk factors are non-modifiable, however smoking is one risk factor that can be modified.

Table 8.4	Risk factors for lupus
Risk factor	**Explanation**
Gender	Women are almost nine times as likely as men to develop lupus
Age	Lupus develops more commonly between the ages of 15 and 45; a woman between these ages is 15 times more likely to develop the disease
Ethnicity	The risk increases in African Americans or Asians
Heredity	It is thought that there is a genetic link
Smoking	Research shows that there is a link between smoking and lupus

RISK OF ANKYLOSING SPONDYLITIS

Although the exact cause of the disease is unknown, research agrees that genetics plays a key role in the development of the disease. It has been found that about 95% of those individuals who have ankylosing spondylitis have a 'genetic marker' called HLA-B27 (this is just a specific protein). It should be noted, however, that individuals who do not have this marker can also develop the disease, and many of those with the marker never develop the disease. Even though HLA-B27 plays a major role in the development of AS, scientists believe that other specific genes are also needed to trigger the disease in susceptible individuals. Having a family history of ankylosing spondylitis also increases the risk of developing the disease, as does having frequent gastrointestinal infections. Gender and age are also considered to be risk factors for this disease. For example, the onset of the disease normally occurs between the ages of 17 and 35 years, however it can affect children and those who are older as well. As far as gender is concerned, the disease is more common in men but it can also affect women.

DIAGNOSIS

The way in which a diagnosis is made across the range of arthritis forms can vary dramatically. For example, in those individuals who display symptoms and might potentially suffer from either osteoarthritis, rheumatoid arthritis or ankylosing spondylitis, a full medical examination including magnetic resonance imaging (an MRI scan, as it is more commonly known) is usually required if X-rays do not provide enough information for a diagnosis to be made. This type of diagnosis has obvious cost implications as specialist equipment is required. To confirm a diagnosis of gout, however, a sample of synovial fluid (the substance that is secreted within a joint for lubrication and protection) is drawn from a suspected inflamed joint (as can be seen in fig 8.4) and examined for uric acid crystals. Even though the cost of this is relatively small, the absence of any uric acid crystals does not completely rule out a diagnosis of the disease, therefore a full case history is usually taken into account before any judgement is made. In the case of lupus there is no single test that can determine whether an individual has the disease or otherwise, but several laboratory tests may help to confirm a diagnosis or at least rule out other causes for an individual's symptoms. Even though

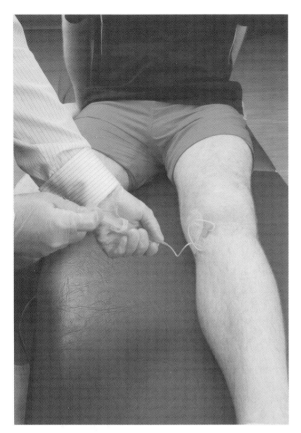

Figure 8.4 Synovial fluid being drawn from the knee

of pain associated with any form of physical activity they might engage in. Unfortunately this often misdirected perception can lead to many problems for the individual, both short and long term, that are associated with inactivity, such as the following:

- loss of flexibility
- muscle atrophy (wastage)
- osteoporosis
- elevated pain threshold
- depression
- fatigue.

The initial objective of undertaking a regular course of physical activity may simply be to reduce the effects associated with inactivity. As far as the benefits of physical activity are concerned, there are several that have commonly been reported, such as improved cardiovascular fitness, muscular fitness and general health status. Generally speaking, research also shows that regular physical activity can improve mood and outlook, and even decrease pain perception. Most people with arthritic diseases are able to participate in regular activities of a gradually progressive nature, even though the starting level may vary greatly between individuals. One of the main goals for this particular population should be to restore normal daily function, prevent further joint damage and restore physical activity levels. It should also be mentioned that there is a range of anti-inflammatory medication that is commonly prescribed for this disease (from aspirin to corticosteroid injections). Fortunately, even though there might be related side effects, physical activity does not interfere with the medication in any way, but vigorous weight-bearing exercises should be avoided for about a week following any

there are blood tests that can be done in order to identify certain autoantibodies that are associated with lupus, a diagnosis can be difficult to make, and it may take a GP or specialist several months or even years to do so.

PHYSICAL ACTIVITY BENEFITS

One of the main concerns for individuals who have arthritis is that of inactivity due to their perception injections that the individual may have had. In relation to osteoarthritis, it is thought that physical activity can help prevent the disease by strengthening the articular cartilage around the ends of bones and also the bone that lies beneath the cartilage (known as subchondral bone). Unfortunately, there is little evidence to show that physical activity can prevent osteoarthritis, although according to Rogers and colleagues in 2002, moderate daily physical activity, especially walking, may be associated with a lower risk, especially among women. It is also generally thought that a broad range of physical activities can help to reduce pain, stiffness and disability, and increase general mobility, gait, function, aerobic fitness and muscle strength. For example, in a study by Ettinger *et al.* in 1997, it was found that three 40-minute walks a week may help to halt the progression of knee osteoarthritis. Physical activity has also been found to help those who have had a joint replacement, even though too much physical activity can be detrimental. For example, according to Stevens *et al.* (2003), if knee osteoarthritis leads to joint replacement, then thigh muscle (quadriceps) strength is often lost and should be addressed after the operation. It has also been suggested by Gilbey and colleagues (2003) that exercise during the periods immediately before and after the operation may help individuals to resume their normal activities more quickly afterwards, as it has been shown that those who have had a joint replacement can recover their aerobic fitness. Caution must be exercised, however, as even though half of joint replacement patients return to walking activities

in the three to nine months after the operation, too much physical activity following the joint replacement can be detrimental, according to McAlindon *et al.* (1999).

PHYSICAL ACTIVITY GUIDELINES

Most forms of arthritis affect the joints, therefore this can influence the individual's capacity to do physical activity. As a general rule, when the disease is at its most painful (i.e. flares up), physical activity levels should be low, even though there is limited research to clarify whether physical activity at this point can further damage the joints affected. It is often reported that, following bouts of physical activity, those with arthritis suffer some degree of discomfort or pain as a result, but the level is dependent on the particular condition of the individual. The length of time for which the discomfort lasts differs as some report the effects lasting several hours and some report effects up to 24 hours later. Finally, it is generally thought that those individuals with arthritis who are not used to participating in regular physical activity have an increased risk of injuries such as sprain, dislocation or fracture as a result of lower bone mineral density in the affected joints. This is potentially as a result of the individual avoiding the use of the joint, which reduces the stress and, over time, reduces bone mineral density. Table 8.5 gives a general overview of physical activity guidelines for those individuals with arthritis.

Table 8.5	Physical activity guidelines for those with arthritis	
	Aerobic training	**Strength training**
Mode	• Walking, cycling and water-based activities are good for this disease	• Focus on joint stability using a range of methods • Start with a small range of movement and build up
Intensity	• Prolonged warm-up and cool-down • 60–80% HRmax depending on the individual • 10–14 RPE	• Use loads within the individual's pain tolerance • Overload by increasing repetitions then intensity
Duration	• 5–30 minutes per session • Increase duration rather than intensity • Multiple short sessions can be done throughout the day	• Perform 1 to 3 sets of 10–15 RM • 1–2 minutes' rest between exercise • Balance major muscle groups and upper/lower body
Frequency	• 3–5 days per week	• 2–3 days per week • Encourage other forms of exercise
Precautions	• Avoid high-impact activities and excessive repetition • If swelling occurs as a result of activity, reduce the intensity and duration • Do activities in the afternoon or evening	• Use isometric exercises on the affected joints • Avoid overstretching • Do not exercise the joint when swollen • Avoid low-carbohydrate diets as this can cause ketosis, leading to increased uric acid concentrations

General precautions
• For all arthritis forms, avoid overrepetition of any activity or exercise.
• If any swelling occurs then reduce the intensity and duration of the activity.
• Do not train any swollen joint.
• Check regularly for any problems with the big toe in cases of gout.
• Focus on mobility during remission of rheumatoid arthritis and ankylosing spondylitis.
• Be aware of warning signs of a lupus flare-up:
  • increased fatigue
  • pain
  • rash
  • fever
  • abdominal discomfort
  • headache
  • dizziness.

RECOMMENDED READING

American College of Sports Medicine (2009a) *ACSM's exercise management for persons with chronic diseases and disabilities* (3rd edn). Champaign, IL: Human Kinetics

American College of Sports Medicine (2009b) *ACSM's guidelines for exercise testing and prescription* (8th edn). London: Lippincott Williams & Wilkins

Benoist, M. (1995) Pierre Marie. Pioneer investigator in ankylosing spondylitis. *Spine*, 20(7): 849–852

Berger, J.W. & Dirk, E.T. (2005) *Andrews' diseases of the skin: Clinical dermatology* (10th edn). Philadelphia, PA: Saunders

Calin, A., Garrett, S., Whitelock, H., Kennedy, L., O'Hea, J., Mallorie, P. & Jenkinson, T. (1994) A new approach to defining functional ability in ankylosing spondylitis: The development of the Bath Ankylosing Spondylitis Functional Index. *Journal of Rheumatology*, 21(12): 2281–2285

Chen, L.X. & Schumacher, H.R. (2008) Gout: An evidence-based review. *Journal of Clinical Rheumatology*, 14(5, suppl.): S55–S62

Choi, H.K., Atkinson, K., Karlson, E.W., Willett, W. & Curhan, G. (2004) Purine-rich foods, dairy and protein intake, and the risk of gout in men. *New England Journal of Medicine*, 350(11): 1093

Department of Health (2004) *At least 5 a week: Evidence on the impact of physical activity and its relationship to health.* London: Department of Health

Ettinger, W.H., Burns, R., Messier, S.P., Applegate, W., Rejeski, W.J., Morgan, T., Shumaker, S. & Berry, M.J. (1997) A randomized trial comparing aerobic exercise and resistance exercise with a health education program in older adults with knee osteoarthritis. The Fitness Arthritis and Seniors Trial (FAST). *Journal of the American Medical Association*, 277(1): 25–31

Firestein, M.D., Gary, S., Budd, M.D., Ralph, C., Harris, M.D. & Edward, D. (eds) (2008) Gout and hyperuricemia. *Kelley's Textbook of Rheumatology* (8th edn). Philadelphia, PA: Elsevier, chapter 87

Gilbey, H.J., Ackland, T.R., Wang, A.W., Morton, A.R., Trouchet, T. & Tapper, J. (2003) Exercise improves early functional recovery after total hip arthroplasty. *Clinical Orthopaedics and Related Research*, 408: 193–200

Gordon, N.F. (1993) *Arthritis: Your complete exercise guide.* Champaign, IL: Human Kinetics

Hak, A.E. & Choi, H.K. (2008) Lifestyle and gout. *Current Opinion in Rheumatology*, 20(2): 179–186

Lueponsak, N., Amin, S., Krebs, D.E., McGibbon, C.A. & Felson, D. (2002) The contribution of type of daily activity to loading across the hip and knee joints in the elderly. *Osteoarthritis and Cartilage*, 10: 353–359

McAlindon, T.E., Wilson, P.W.F., Aliabadi, P., Weissman, B. & Felson, D.T. (1999) Level of physical activity and the risk of radiographic and symptomatic knee osteoarthritis in the elderly: The Framingham Study. *American Journal of Medicine*, 106: 151–157

Padyukov, L., Silva, C., Stolt, P., Alfredsson, L. & Klareskog, L. (2004) A gene-environment interaction between smoking and shared epitope genes in HLA-DR provides a high risk of seropositive rheumatoid arthritis. *Arthritis Rheumatology*, 50: 3085–3092

Pope, D.P., Hunt, I.M., Birrell, F.N., Siulman, A.J. & MacFarlane, G.J. (2003) Hip pain onset in relation to cumulative workplace and leisure time mechanical load: A population based case control study. *Annals of the Rheumatic Diseases*, 62: 322–326

Rogers, L.Q., Macera, C.A., Hootman, J.M., Ainsworth, B.E. & Blair, S.N. (2002) The association between joint stress from physical activity and self-reported osteoarthritis: An analysis of the Cooper Clinic data. *Osteoarthritis and Cartilage*, 10: 617–622

Stevens, J.E., Mizner, R.L. & Snyder-Mackler, L. (2003) Quadriceps strength and volitional activation before and after total knee arthroplasty for osteoarthritis. *Journal of Orthopaedic Research*, 21: 775–779

Terkeltaub, R. (2010) Update on gout: New therapeutic strategies and options. *National Reviews in Rheumatology*, 6(1): 30–38

Thorburn, C.M., Prokunina-Olsson, L., Sterba, K.A., Lum, R.F., Seldin, M.F., Alarcón-Riquelme, M.E. & Criswell, L.A. (2007) Association of PDCD1 genetic variation with risk and clinical manifestations of systemic lupus erythematosus in a multiethnic cohort. *Genes Immunology*, 8: 279–287

Williams, P.T. (2008) Effects of diet, physical activity and performance, and body weight on incident gout in ostensibly healthy, vigorously active men. *American Journal of Clinical Nutrition*, 87(5): 1480–1487

USEFUL WEBSITES

Arthritis Research UK – www.arthritisresearchuk.org
Department of Health – www.dh.gov.uk
National Institute of Arthritis and Musculoskeletal and
    Skin Diseases – www.niams.nih.gov

// OSTEOPOROSIS

9

KEYPOINTS

- Osteoporosis is a condition of the bones that increases the risk of fracture or break due to loss of bone mass.
- The loss of bone mass tends to occur earlier in women than it does in men.
- The loss of bone mass can be accelerated for a period up to five years post-menopause.
- Figures show that one in three women and one in twelve men, over the age of 50 years, in the UK will sustain a spine, hip or wrist fracture due to the condition of osteoporosis.
- Approximately one in three over-65s and 50% of over-85s fall each year.
- Physical activity can increase bone mineral density in adolescents, maintain it in young adults and slow its decline in old age.
- For optimal protection against osteoporosis, activity that physically stresses bones, such as running, jumping, skipping, gymnastics or jogging, is recommended.
- Physical activity in later life can delay the progression of osteoporosis, but it cannot reverse advanced bone loss.
- Physical activity programmes can help reduce the risk of falling, and therefore fractures, among older people.

WHAT IS IT?

In simple terms, osteoporosis is a condition of the bones that increases the risk of fracture or break. In the early 19th century, a distinguished English surgeon by the name of Sir Astley Paston Cooper reported that the lightness and softness that bones acquired in the more advanced stages of life favoured the production of fractures, meaning that the older we get the higher the risk of bone fracture. The term osteoporosis, however, was first used by the pathologist and surgeon Johann Lobstein at about the same time, in which he attributed the condition to a loss of calcium. Then, in 1940, an American endocrinologist by the name of Fuller Albright described the condition of post-menopausal (after the menopause) osteoporosis and proposed that it was the consequence of impaired bone formation due to oestrogen (female hormone) deficiency in women. Even though this seems to suggest that there are two main forms of osteoporosis, current thinking is that there are many mechanisms that can cause loss of bone mass and deterioration of the skeletal structure. Osteoporosis is more common as we get older, as is the increased risk of falls, which is why there is a much higher incidence of fragility fractures in osteoporotic individuals as there is in non-osteoporotic individuals. Research over the years has shown that generally from about the age of 35 years all humans are prone to losing bone mass (although the loss can be very small in many cases) due to the inactivity of bone-forming cells in the body. The amount of bone loss can vary substantially due to many individual differences such as physical activity levels, dietary habits and many other factors. Unfortunately, it is commonly recognised that an increase in bone mass loss is related to an increase in risk of bone fracture. When bone fractures occur in situations that are considered to be 'minimal trauma' and are as a result of having low bone mass, the condition is then referred to as 'osteoporosis'. In terms of gender difference, many recent statistics show that osteoporosis is more common in women than it is in men (it is three times more common in women than in men) after women have reached the age of menopause. The cause of osteoporosis can be complex and is not yet fully understood; it can often be difficult to diagnose as some sufferers do not realise that they have osteoporosis until late into the condition. There are both modifiable and non-modifiable causes related to osteoporosis; those considered to be the main ones are outlined in table 9.1.

PREVALENCE

It is evident that, on a global scale, the loss of bone mass (as discussed earlier) generally occurs earlier in women than it does in men. This bone mass loss can also be accelerated for a period up to five years post-menopause (this is thought to be linked

Table 9.1	Potential causes of osteoporosis
Potential cause	**Description**
Hormonal disorder	This may occur in anyone with a particular hormonal disorder, such as those with a disease of the parathyroid glands, which leads to a condition known as hyperparathyroidism
Medication induced	The condition may occur as a result of certain medications such as glucocorticoids; if this occurs it is known as steroid or glucocorticoid-induced osteoporosis (SIOP or GIOP)
Menopause	In females, a disruption of hormone balance as a result of menopause can be a major cause of osteoporosis
Diet	Over-consumption of dietary protein is also related to osteoporosis; the excess protein causes calcium to be taken from the bones and excreted in the urine

to the reduction of oestrogen levels in women). According to an investigation carried out by Van Staa and colleagues in 2001, figures show that in the UK about one in two women and one in five men, over the age of 50 years, will sustain a spine, hip or wrist fracture mainly as a result of osteoporosis. This is quite an important statistic considering there are almost 20 million people in the UK over the age of 50. Even though fractures can occur anywhere in the body, those in the area of the hip are considered to have the greatest effect. For example, research by Todd *et al.* (1995) has shown that 18% of those individuals in the UK who suffer a hip fracture, die within three months of the injury. This figure is extremely high as a reported 30% of adults over the age of 65 years suffer a fall each year. As a result of the high prevalence of hospitalised cases, the burden on the NHS is enormous. One example of this can be seen in a report by Burge in the *Journal of Medical*

Economics in 2001, where it was estimated that, by 2020, the cost of treating all osteoporotic fractures in post-menopausal women would be more than £2.1 billion.

SYMPTOMS

Osteoporosis is sometimes known as the 'silent epidemic' as there are no specific or obvious symptoms or warning signs until late in the condition when a bone fracture normally occurs. Severe cases of osteoporosis can result in an upper-body postural problem known as 'kyphosis'. This problem can easily be seen as an individual has a hunched posture and the upper back area is rounded and hump-like, as can be seen in fig 9.1. There can be several associated problems in cases where an individual has a kyphotic posture. For example, respiratory function can be impaired as

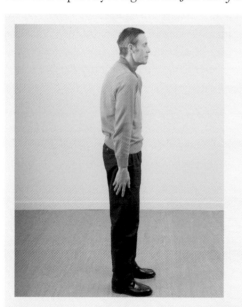 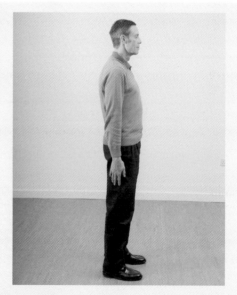

Figure 9.1 Typical kyphotic posture compared to good posture

the lung space and chest cavity is often compressed. Another problem is that the risk of falling can be increased due to the centre of gravity being moved forward, making the individual more unstable. As very frail bone structures are considered a typical indication of this condition, resultant repeated bone fractures are a very common occurrence, especially when they happen with little or no apparent trauma to the site of injury. The most frequent sites for osteoporotic-type fractures are the vertebrae, wrist and hip.

bone mineral density throughout their lives, especially around the time of the growth spurt (which occurs at about 12 years in girls and 14 years in boys). In the case of both males and females, those who reach puberty at a later stage tend to have lower bone mineral densities. Possibly the worst combination for reduced bone mass in women is when menstruation starts late and the individual also suffers an early menopause (the average female menopause being about 51 years of age).

RISK FACTORS

Regardless of the extent of bone mass loss that different individuals may experience, there are several commonly cited risk factors that are considered to be related to osteoporosis. Some of these are classed as 'non-modifiable' in that nothing can be done to reduce or eliminate the potential risk, whereas others are classed as 'modifiable' as it is agreed that some sort of intervention can be made in order to reduce the risk (see table 9.2).

Although nothing can be done about this particular event, ageing is considered to be one of the main risk factors for the development of osteoporosis. Both males and females rapidly gain

DIAGNOSIS

Even though a good indication of osteoporosis can simply be the number and frequency of fractures sustained, along with a visual sighting of a individual's posture and frame, a clinical diagnosis as a result of specific testing can also be made. Radiography, computerised tomography (CT) and magnetic resonance imaging (MRI) scans are all clinical testing methods that are often used to build up a picture of the bone state of the individual. Measuring bone mineral density (BMD) is another method that can be used. The most popular method of measuring BMD is dual-energy X-ray absorptiometry (DEXA). This is a method that is often considered to be the gold

Table 9.2 Non-modifiable and modifiable risk factors for osteoporosis	
Non-modifiable	**Modifiable**
Female	Inactivity
Older age	Excessive smoking
Caucasian or Asian	Excessive alcohol (more than 2 units per day)
Family history	Low dietary calcium and vitamin D
Premature menopause	Prolonged amenorrhea* (loss of periods)

* It is sometimes possible to modify this problem, for example when the case of overtraining is the cause.

standard for clinically diagnosing osteoporosis. It should be noted that clinical testing and diagnosis should be carried out only by appropriately qualified people.

PHYSICAL ACTIVITY BENEFITS

There is much evidence available to show that physical activity can slow and in some cases halt the decline in bone mass. There is however very little evidence to show that physical activity can reverse the effects of the condition even though some reports have claimed a 5% increase in bone mass as a result of a combination of regular physical activity and calcium supplements. According to the Department of Health (2004), physical activity that places stress on bone (such as running, jumping and skipping) can increase bone mineral density in adolescents, maintain it in young adults and slow its decline in old age. This has also been shown in research such as in the investigation by Vuori in 2001. This particular investigation highlighted that the effect was greatest in the bones that were most heavily loaded during the physical activities that were undertaken. In another investigation, by Welten and colleagues (1994), it was also pointed out that it is important to increase bone mineral density in adolescents, because this reduces the chances of loss of bone mass later in life, which subsequently reduces the risk of bone fracture as well. In terms of the amount of activity needed, in a study by Cooper et al. (1998), it was suggested that doing more than 5 hours of physical activity a week was best for reducing the risk of hip fracture. The main point and consensus of the majority of research in

this area is that regular physical activity undertaken into the mid-20s is essential to help develop bone mass. It has been shown regularly in studies such as that by Snow et al. in 2000, that when an individual reaches adulthood, regular physical activity can help to slow down the rate of bone loss. It has even been suggested that some bone gain might still be possible as a result of physical activity (although this is a topic of much debate). Snow et al. also suggested in their research that physical activity may help to regulate the production and circulation of certain hormones, and also improve balance ability. These claims have also been supported by other studies such as that with previously inactive women aged 65–75 years. This particular investigation consisted of 20 weeks of twice-weekly physical activity classes, which resulted in improved dynamic balance and strength. In terms of improving strength and power, research such as that by Foldvari et al. in 2000 has shown that this is also possible in older adults. This improvement in strength and power is important as it can help to prevent up to 25% of falls as, according to the American and British Geriatrics societies, muscle weakness is the strongest risk factor for falling. This has been supported by other community studies such as those by Hogan et al. (2001) and Chang et al. (2004), which show that physical activity programmes can reduce rates of falling.

PHYSICAL ACTIVITY GUIDELINES

Many current recommendations are for physical activity programmes that include both aerobic and muscle-strengthening physical activities. Many older individuals will be deconditioned, therefore programmes should start with only a few minutes of aerobic training and gradually build up to longer periods, or intersperse aerobic activity with resistance exercises. Strength training is important in order to help maintain levels of bone mass, and to help improve dynamic balance (balance when moving) and reduce the risk of falling. This is extremely important, as research by Youm and colleagues (1999) has shown that about 90% of all hip fractures, which are considered to be the most traumatic of all fractures, are caused by falling, and the falls are more than likely due to lack of muscular strength. As strength training mainly affects the areas that are specifically targeted by

the exercises used, programmes should always try to incorporate both upper- and lower-body muscle groups as well as left and right sides, in order to create muscle balance in the body. It is likely (and recommended) that anyone supervising individuals with osteoporosis would work in conjunction with a physician and physical therapist as the initial assessment and programming of a regular physical activity routine is of paramount importance. However, for those individuals with milder forms of the condition, there are general physical activity guidelines that could be followed (see table 9.3) to allow supervisors a degree of independence.

Table 9.3 Physical activity guidelines for people with osteoporosis

	Aerobic training	Strength training
Mode	• Walking, cycling and water-based physical activity is better for those with reduced tolerance for weight bearing	• As well as strength, include mobility physical activities • Focus on the vulnerable areas susceptible to fracture
Intensity	• Work to maximal limits as tolerated by symptoms of the individual	• Use light weights to start • Overload by increasing repetitions then intensity
Duration	• 20–30 minutes per session • Increase physical activity duration rather than intensity • Slow progression	• Perform 2 to 3 sets of 12–15 RM • 1–2 minutes' rest between physical activities
Frequency	• 3–5 days per week	• 2–3 days per week • Encourage other forms of physical activity
Precautions	• Constantly monitor feedback using pain and RPE scales • Only include impact if it can be tolerated	• Avoid muscular fatigue • Balance upper and lower body • Don't forget to work on posture and balance

General precautions
• See table 9.4

Table 9.4	Physical activity precautions for people with osteoporosis
Precaution	**Comment**
In most cases forward flexion of the spine (bending forward from the waist) should be avoided, or at least limited	Forward flexion may increase the risk of new fractures
Avoid lying on the front and back; choose seated or standing alternatives	Those susceptible to vertebral fractures will be more at risk with lying down
Limit the amount of weight-bearing physical activities at the start, and progress slowly	If weight-bearing physical activities cause pain, alternative water-based activities should be given
Do not overestimate fitness levels	Individuals in this population tend to be less fit than the average population as a result of the decreased mobility
Always stay close to the client during all physical activities	Individuals in this population also tend to have a fear of falling and those with excessive lean may be unstable
Recommend a good nutritional strategy to complement the physical activity programme	Nutritional status can play a major role in this condition

Due to the fragile nature of this condition there are several precautions (see table 9.4) that should be taken when working with those suffering from osteoporosis, regardless of the severity.

Once osteoporosis has been diagnosed there are several medication treatments commonly prescribed. Hormone replacement therapy (HRT) is the most common and is used to replace hormone levels post-menopause. This has the effect of slowing down bone remodelling. Other prescribed medications include calcitonin, bisphosphonates and sodium fluoride.

RECOMMENDED READING

American College of Sports Medicine (2009a) *ACSM's exercise management for persons with chronic diseases and disabilities* (3rd edn). Champaign, IL: Human Kinetics

American College of Sports Medicine (2009b) *ACSM's guidelines for exercise testing and prescription* (8th edn). London: Lippincott Williams & Wilkins

American Geriatric Society, British Geriatric Society, American Academy of Orthopedic Surgeons Panel on Falls Prevention (2001) Guidelines for the prevention of falls in older people. *Journal of the American Geriatrics Society*, 49: 664–672

Berg, K.M., Kunins, H.V., Jackson, J.L., Nahvi, S., Chaudhry, A., Harris, K.A., Malik, R. & Arnsten, J.H. (2008) Association between alcohol consumption and both osteoporotic fracture and bone density. *American Journal of Medicine*, 121(5): 406–418

Bonaiuti, D., Shea, B., Iovine, R., Negrini, S., Welch, V., Kemper H.H.G.C., Wells, G.A., Tugwell, P. & Cranney, A. (2002) Physical activity for preventing and treating osteoporosis in post-menopausal women. *Cochrane Database of Systematic Reviews*, 2: CD 000333

Bone and Tooth Society of Great Britain, National Osteoporosis Society, Royal College of Physicians (2002) *Glucocorticoid-induced osteoporosis*. London: Royal College of Physicians of London. London: The Lavenham Press

Burge, R.T. (2001) The cost of osteoporotic fractures in the UK. Projections for 2000–2020. *Journal of Medical Economics*, 4: 51–62

Chang, J.T., Morton, S.C., Rubenstein, L.Z., Mojica, W.A., Maglione, M., Suttorp, M.J., Roth, E.A. & Shekelle, P.G. (2004) Interventions for the prevention of falls in older adults: Systematic review and meta-analysis of randomised clinical trials. *British Medical Journal*, 328: 680

Chien, M.Y., Wu, Y.T., Hsu, A.T., Yang, R.S. & Lai, J.S. (2000) Efficacy of a 24-week aerobic physical activity program for osteopenic post-menopausal women. *Calcified Tissue International*, 67(6): 443–448

Cooper, C., Barker, D.J. & Wickham, C. (1998) Physical activity, muscle strength and calcium intake in fracture of the proximal femur in Britain. *British Medical Journal*, 297: 1443–1446

Dalsky, G.P., Stocke, K.S., Ehsani, A.A., Slatopolsky, E., Lee, W.C. & Birge, S.J. (1988) Weight-bearing physical activity training and lumbar bone mineral content in post-menopausal women. *Annals of Internal Medicine*, 108(6): 824–828

Davis, S., Sachdeva, A., Goeckeritz, B. & Oliver, A. (2010) All about osteoporosis: A comprehensive analysis. *Journal of Musculoskeletal Medicine*, 27(4): 149–153

Department of Health (2004) *At least 5 a week: Evidence on the impact of physical activity and its relationship to health*. London: Department of Health

DIPART (vitamin D Individual Patient Analysis of Randomized Trials) (2010) Patient level pooled analysis of 68 500 patients from seven major vitamin D fracture trials in US and Europe. *British Medical Journal*, 340: B5463

Ebeling, P.R. (2008) Clinical practice. Osteoporosis in men. *New England Journal of Medicine*, 358(14): 1474–1482

Foldvari, M., Clark, M., Laviolette, L.C., Bernstein, M.A., Kaliton, D., Castaneda, C., Pu, C.T., Hausdorff, J.M., Fielding, R.A. & Singh, M.A. (2000) Association of muscle power with functional status in community-dwelling elderly women. *Journals of Gerontology Series A, Biological Sciences and Medical Sciences*, 55: M192–M199

Ganz, D.A., Bao, Y., Shekelle, P.G. & Rubenstein, L.Z. (2007) Will my patient fall? *Journal of the American Medical Association*, 297(1): 77–86

Guglielmi, G. & Scalzo, G. (2010) Imaging tools transform diagnosis of osteoporosis. *Diagnostic Imaging Europe*, 26(3): 7–11

Hogan, D.B., MacDonald, F.A., Betts, J., Bricker, S., Ebly, E.M., Delarue, B., Fung, T.S., Harbidge, C., Hunter, M., Maxwell, C.J. & Metcalf, B. (2001) A randomized controlled trial of a community-based consultation service to prevent falls. *Canadian Medical Association Journal*, 165: 537–543

Ilich, J.Z. & Kerstetter, J.E. (2000) Nutrition in bone health revisited: A story beyond calcium. *Journal of the American College of Nutrition*, 19(6): 715–737

Poole, K.E. & Compston, J.E. (2006) Osteoporosis and its management. *British Medical Journal*, 333(7581): 1251–1256

Raisz, L. (2005) Pathogenesis of osteoporosis: Concepts, conflicts, and prospects. *Journal of Clinical Investigation*, 115(12): 3318–3325

Riggs, B.L. & Melton, L.J. (1988) *Osteoporosis: Etiology, diagnosis and management*. New York: Raven Press

Shapses, S.A. & Riedt, C.S. (2006) Bone, body weight, and weight reduction: What are the concerns? *Journal of Nutrition*, 136(6): 1453–1456

Sinaki, M., Brey, R.H., Hughes, C.A., Larson, D.R. & Kaufman, K.R. (2005) Significant reduction in risk of falls and back pain in osteoporotic-kyphotic women through a Spinal Proprioceptive Extension Physical Activity Dynamic (SPEED) program. *Mayo Clinic Proceedings*, 80(7): 849–855

Snow, C.M., Shaw, J.M., Winters, K.M. & Witzke, K.A. (2000) Long-term physical activity using weighted vests prevents hip bone loss in post-menopausal women. *Journals of Gerontology Series A, Biological Sciences and Medical Sciences*, 55: M489–M491

Todd, C.J., Freeman, C.J., Camilleri-Ferrante, C., Palmer, C.R., Hyder, A., Laxton, C.E., Parker, M.J., Payne, B.V. & Rushton, N. (1995) Differences in mortality after fracture of hip: The East Anglian audit. *British Medical Journal*, 310: 904–908

Van Staa, T.P., Dennison, E.M., Leufkens, H.G. & Cooper, C. (2001) Epidemiology of fractures in England and Wales. *Bone*, 29: 517–522

Vuori, I.M. (2001) Dose-response of physical activity and low back pain, osteoarthritis, and osteoporosis. *Medicine and Science in Sports and Physical Activity*, 33: S551–S586

Waugh, E.J., Lam, M.A, Hawker, G.A., McGowan, J., Papaioannou, A., Cheung, A.M., Hodsman, A.B., Leslie, W.D., Siminoski, K. & Jamal, S.A. (2009) Risk factors for low bone mass in healthy 40–60-year-old women: A systematic review of the literature. *Osteoporosis International*, 20(1): 1–21

Welten, D.C., Kemper, H.C., Post, G.B., Van Mechelen, W., Twisk, J., Lips, P. & Teule, G.J. (1994) Weight-bearing activity during youth is a more important factor for peak bone mass than calcium intake. *Journal of Bone and Mineral Research*, 9: 1089–1096

Wong, P.K., Christie, J.J. & Wark, J.D. (2007) The effects of smoking on bone health. *Clinical Science*, 113(5): 233–241

World Health Organization (2002) *Report of a Joint WHO/FAO/UNU Expert Consultation: Protein and amino acid requirements in human nutrition*. Geneva, Switzerland: WHO Press

World Health Organization (2003) *WHO Technical Report Series 921. Prevention and management of osteoporosis: Report of a WHO scientific group*. Geneva, Switzerland: WHO Press

Youm, T., Koval, K.J., Kummer, F.J. & Zuckerman, J.D. (1999) Do all hip fractures result from a fall? *American Journal of Orthopedics*, 28: 190–194

USEFUL WEBSITES

American Academy of Orthopaedic Surgeons – www.aaos.org

American Geriatrics Society – www.americangeriatrics.org

Bone Research Society – www.brsoc.org.uk

British Geriatrics Society – www.bgs.org.uk

Department of Health – www.dh.gov.uk

National Osteoporosis Society – www.nos.org.uk

Royal College of Physicians – www.rcplondon.ac.uk

World Health Organization – www.who.int/en

PARKINSON'S DISEASE

10

KEYPOINTS

- The Parkinson's Disease Society estimates that there are about 120,000 individuals in the UK with the disease.
- Approximately 10,000 individuals are diagnosed with the disease each year.
- About 20% of Parkinson's disease patients have at least one relative with symptoms, suggesting that a genetic factor may be involved.
- Most researchers believe that most cases are not caused by genetic factors alone.
- According to the National Collaborating Centre for Chronic Conditions there are more males with the disease and the direct costs of treatment to the NHS have been estimated at approximately £2298 per patient per year.
- Physical activity is effective in the treatment of clinical depression and can be as successful as psychotherapy or medication.
- Physical activity can help individuals with anxiety, phobias, panic attacks and stress.
- Physical activity can have a positive effect on well-being; it can also help individuals feel better about themselves through improved physical self-perceptions, and can improve self-esteem, particularly in those with initial low self-esteem.
- It is recommended that anyone who wishes to supervise activity for someone with Parkinson's disease always liaise with a physiotherapist or other health professional before they do so if they lack the experience or feel that they are not sufficiently confident.
- The main goal of any physical activity programme should be to increase the capacity of the individual to perform daily living activities.

WHAT IS IT?

Parkinson's disease (PD) is often classed as a chronic, progressive neurodegenerative movement disorder. In other words, the disease, is related to movement problems that get worse steadily over time. This is not a recent disease, as symptoms of Parkinson's have been known and treated since medieval times. However, it was not formally documented until 1817 in 'An essay on the shaking palsy' by a physician called James Parkinson, hence the condition became known as Parkinson's disease (even though there are different classifications of the disease). In the most common classification, which is when the cause is unknown, the disease is referred to as 'idiopathic Parkinson's'. There are other forms of Parkinson's disease in which a cause is known or suspected, but these represent a very small percentage of overall cases. The cause of Parkinson's disease is thought to result from the degeneration of certain nerve cells in the brain, which are dopamine-producing nerve cells. When dopamine (a neurotransmitter) production is reduced, or even depleted, the motor system nerves (or motor neurons, as they are known) are unable to control movement and coordination. The depletion of dopamine is depicted in fig 10.1.

It is unfortunate, but those people with Parkinson's disease have normally lost about 80% or more of their dopamine-producing cells by the time any symptoms appear. Even though the cause of Parkinson's disease is largely unknown, some researchers believe that several factors may be involved, such as free radicals, accelerated ageing, environmental toxins and genetic predisposition. As far as free radicals are

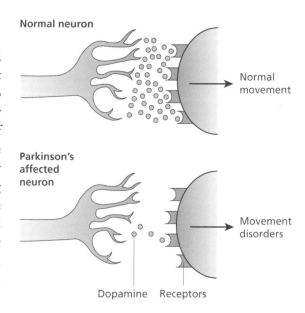

Figure 10.1 Dopamine levels from a normal cell and cell affected by PD

concerned, it is thought that they may be involved in the degeneration of dopamine-producing cells as they are highly chemically reactive charged particles. Exposure to an environmental toxin, such as a pesticide, that inhibits dopamine production is just one way that free radicals can be produced in the body. Smoking and certain dietary factors are just some of the alternative means of producing free radicals. It is widely known that eating foods with high levels of antioxidants, such as those that are high in vitamins A, C and E, are good for combating the effects of free radicals. Many types of fruit and vegetables are good sources of these vitamins, which is just one of the reasons why a varied diet that highlights the government's five-a-day message is recommended at a population level.

PREVALENCE

The Parkinson's Disease Society estimates that there are about 120,000 individuals in the UK at any one time with the disease (1 in 500 of the general population), and that approximately 10,000 new cases are diagnosed each year. About 20% of those diagnosed with Parkinson's disease have at least one relative with symptoms, leading researchers to suggest that genetic factors may be involved. Most researchers do believe, however, that the majority of cases are not caused by genetic factors alone. According to the National Collaborating Centre for Chronic Conditions, there are more males than there are females with the disease, and the direct costs of treatment to the NHS have been estimated to be approximately £2298 per patient per year.

SYMPTOMS

The many symptoms of Parkinson's disease may appear at any age, but the average age of onset of the actual disease is normally around 60 years. Most individuals with Parkinson's disease do not develop all of the symptoms associated with the disease and can in some cases develop only one. Symptoms also vary in that they may progress quickly or gradually over years, depending on the individual case. Those individuals who have been diagnosed with idiopathic Parkinson's disease often develop several of the symptoms (which may vary from day to day) over a period of time, but they typically develop some of the primary symptoms (see table 10.1 for a description) such as bradykinesia, tremor, rigidity, postural and balance problems, and Parkinsonian gait.

Table 10.1	Primary symptoms of Parkinson's disease
Primary symptom	**Description**
Bradykinesia	Slowness and unpredictable involuntary movement; difficulty initiating movement, as well as difficulty completing movement once it is in progress; everyday activities that could previously be carried out easily (such as bathing or dressing) could take hours
Tremors	Tremor is the primary symptom for some patients, but only a minor complaint for others; the tremor is normally a rhythmic back-and-forth motion of the thumb and forefinger at three beats per second; this is sometimes called 'pill rolling'; tremor mainly begins in a hand and is most obvious when at rest; in the early stages, in 75% of patients the tremor usually affects one side of the body, becoming more generalised in later stages
Rigidity	Rigidity is the term used for increased muscular resistance to movement; in this condition, the muscles remain constantly tensed and contracted so that they ache and feel stiff and weak
Poor posture and balance	Poor balance and coordination often causes patients to lean forwards or backwards and to fall easily; if bumped or when starting to walk, sufferers who lean backwards tend to step backwards (known as retropulsion); poor posture can develop, such as hunched shoulders and dropped head
Parkinsonian gait	This is the distinctive unsteady walk associated with Parkinson's disease, often with a series of quick, small steps known as festination; also, the arms swing only a little or not at all

Table 10.2	Secondary symptoms of Parkinson's disease
Secondary symptoms	**Description**
Dysphagia	Difficulty swallowing saliva, and food that collects in the mouth or back of the throat may cause choking, coughing or drooling
Hypersalivation	Many suffer from excessive salivation
Hyperhidrosis	The disease often causes excessive sweating
Cognitive changes	Loss of intellectual capacity; those with PD have a sixfold increased risk of getting dementia; depression may also appear – it might not be severe, but it may be intensified by the drugs used to treat other symptoms of PD
Seborrhoea	This is scaling, dry skin on the face and scalp, and oily skin on the forehead and at the sides of the nose
Micrographia	Sufferers often have small, cramped handwriting
Dysarthria	About 50% of all PD patients have problems with speech, such as speaking softly (hypophonia), hesitating, slurring or repeating their words, or speaking too fast
Other	Obsessive-compulsive behaviour such as binge eating and craving; loss of bladder and/or bowel control; loss of facial expression

As well as the primary symptoms that are described in table 10.1, there are also many other symptoms that are associated with Parkinson's disease, known as secondary symptoms. A range of secondary symptoms, adapted from various sources, is described in table 10.2.

It is also interesting to note that this particular disease is linked to several other health-related conditions. For example, it is estimated that over 20% of individuals who have Parkinson's disease also develop another condition known as 'dementia', which results in a serious loss of cognitive ability. It is also estimated that about 50% of all individuals who have Parkinson's disease suffer from some degree of depression.

RISK FACTORS

Much research is still in progress regarding the risk factors associated with Parkinson's disease. Generally it is thought that there is no single main factor but rather an accumulation of factors. These can range from exposures to certain toxins, ageing of the central nervous system (CNS) or other cell death mechanisms. It is known that genetic factors may also play a role, particularly if the disease begins before the age of 50. There is a relatively new line of research in linking the role of genetic factors to the development of the disease, as it has been shown that about 15–20% of those with Parkinson's have a close relative who has experienced Parkinsonian symptoms, such as a tremor.

DIAGNOSIS

Common symptoms of the disease are often easily identified, however it can be difficult to diagnose accurately as there is no consistently reliable test that can distinguish the disease from other conditions that have similar clinical presentations. For this reason, a full diagnosis is always carried out by appropriately qualified individuals and is generally based on a combination of identifying certain symptoms and ruling out other disorders that produce similar symptoms. A neurological exam and medical history, followed by a computerised tomography (CT) scan or magnetic resonance imaging (MRI) scan is sometimes done to rule out other disorders (e.g. brain tumour, stroke) that produce Parkinsonian symptoms. There are, however, well-known diagnostic criteria tests that have been widely adopted in the UK, such as the criteria from the UK Parkinson's Disease Society Brain Bank and those from the National Institute of Neurological Disorders and Stroke. For example, the UK Parkinson's Disease Society Brain Bank has the diagnostic criteria listed in the text box.

PHYSICAL ACTIVITY BENEFITS

Unfortunately there is limited research in the area of benefits of physical activity for those with Parkinson's disease. It is generally thought, however, that regular physical activity can have a range of benefits in reducing the effect of some of the symptoms, such as the following:

- increased cardiovascular fitness
- prevention of joint deformity
- improved joint mobility
- improved coordination and balance
- increased muscle strength and flexibility
- reduced muscle cramping
- improved posture
- improved control over gross motor movements, such as walking
- reduced stress levels
- greater confidence in performing daily activities.

Even though it is generally considered that regular physical activity cannot halt the progression of Parkinson's disease, according to research

Test box: UK Parkinson's Disease Society Brain Bank criteria

Note: This is a clinical diagnosis only.
1   In the first instance the individual must suffer from slowness of movement (bradykinesia) and either rigidity, rest tremor or postural instability.
2   Second, other possible causes for symptoms have to be ruled out.
3   Next, the individual would have to have three or more of the following during onset or evolution: unilateral onset, rest tremor, progression, asymmetry of motor symptoms, response to levodopa during at least five years, clinical course of at least ten years and appearance of dyskinesias (movement disorders) induced by the intake of excessive levodopa.

presented at the American Academy of Neurology's 59th Annual Meeting in Boston in April and May 2007, the risk of developing Parkinson's disease may be reduced with a regular programme of moderate to vigorous exercise or other specific recreational activities.

PHYSICAL ACTIVITY GUIDELINES

It is recommended that anyone who wishes to supervise activity for someone with Parkinson's disease always liaise with a physiotherapist or other health professional before they do so if they lack experience or feel that they are not sufficiently confident. The main goal of any physical activity programme should be to increase the capacity of the individual to perform daily living activities.

As can be seen in the guidelines in table 10.3, a balance trainer is a recommended tool for Parkinson's disease. This is a piece of equipment that is commonly available and can be used with many different types of population (see fig 10.2). Many gyms and fitness centres now have this equipment as it is proving to be extremely popular.

Table 10.3	Physical activity guidelines for those individuals with Parkinson's disease	
	Aerobic training	**Strength training**
Mode	• Aerobic such as leg and arm cycle ergometry* and rowing • Short walking bouts of 20–30 m	• Focus on maintaining strength of arms, shoulders, legs and hips • Balance trainers are a good tool to use
Intensity	• 60–85%HRmax • 10–15 RPE	• Use loads within the individual's capability • Overload by increasing repetitions then intensity
Duration	• 15–20 minutes per session or 4–6 sessions per day	• Perform 1 set of 8–12 RM
Frequency	• 3 days per week	• 3 sessions per week • Encourage other forms of exercise
Precautions	• Stop and rest if tired at any point as overexertion can make symptoms worse	• Make sure good posture is maintained • Do not forget functional movements

General precautions
- Include a warm-up and cool-down.
- Include a thorough stretching routine that targets each joint and muscle group.
- Maintain capacity to perform as many daily living activities as possible.
- Be aware that individuals may have balance problems.

* An 'ergometer' is the name given to a machine that can measure the amount of work being done.

In terms of using the equipment, an individual stands on the footplate of the balance trainer, which can be set to pivot with different levels of responsiveness. This means that the individual has to control the movement of the footplate in order to keep it level and balanced. This can be useful for those just wishing to improve balance ability or those recovering from orthopaedic injury. Most balance trainers also have various built-in tests that can be done at different levels to cater for progression. Some of the tests can also give an overall indication of balance ability, which is displayed as a fall-risk rating.

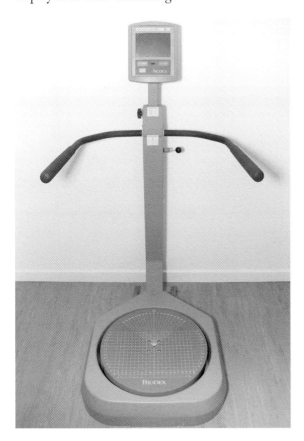

Figure 10.2 A typical balance trainer

RECOMMENDED READING

American College of Sports Medicine (2009a) *ACSM's exercise management for persons with chronic diseases and disabilities* (3rd edn). Champaign, IL: Human Kinetics

American College of Sports Medicine (2009b) *ACSM's guidelines for exercise testing and prescription* (8th edn). London: Lippincott Williams & Wilkins

British Brain and Spine Foundation (1998) *Parkinson's disease and Parkinsonism: A guide for patients and carers.* London: British Brain and Spine Foundation

Brooks, D.J. (2010) Imaging approaches to Parkinson disease. *Journal of Nuclear Medicine*, 51(4): 596–609

Caballol, N., Martí, M.J. & Tolosa, E. (2007) Cognitive dysfunction and dementia in Parkinson disease. *Movement Disorders*, 22(17): S358–S366

Chade, A.R., Kasten, M. & Tanner, C.M. (2006) Nongenetic causes of Parkinson's disease. *Journal of Neural Transmission*, 70(suppl.): 147–151

Davie, C.A. (2008) A review of Parkinson's disease. *British Medical Bulletin*, 86: 109–127

Gelb, D.J., Oliver, E. & Gilman, S. (1999) Diagnostic criteria for Parkinson disease. *Archives of Neurology*, 56: 33–39

Goldenberg, M.M. (2008) Medical management of Parkinson's disease. *Pharmacy and Therapeutics*, 33(10): 590–606

Goodwin, V.A., Richards, S.H., Taylor, R.S., Taylor, A.H. & Campbell, J.L. (2008) The effectiveness of exercise interventions for individuals with Parkinson's disease: A systematic review and meta-analysis. *Movement Disorders*, 23(5): 631–640

Hardy, J., Cookson, M.R. & Singleton, A. (2003) Genes and parkinsonism. *Lancet Neurology*, 2: 221–228

Howard Hughes Medical Institute (2006) Parkinson's disease mechanism discovered, 22 June. Available online at: www.hhmi.org/news/lindquist20060622.html (accessed 20 July 2010)

Jankovic, J. (2008) Parkinson's disease: Clinical features and diagnosis. *Journal of Neurology, Neurosurgery and Psychiatry*, 79(4): 368–376

Klein, C., Pramstaller, P.P., Kis, B., Page, C.C., Kann, M., Leung, J., Woodward, H., Castellan, C.C., Scherer, M., Vieregge, P., Breakefield, X.O., Kramer, P.L. &

Ozelius, L.J. (2000) Parkin deletions in a family with adult-onset, tremor-dominant parkinsonism: Expanding the phenotype. *Annals of Neurology*, 48: 65–71

Lee, M.S. & Ernst, E. (2009) Qigong for movement disorders: A systematic review. *Movement Disorders*, 24(2): 301–303

Lee, M.S., Lam, P. & Ernst, E. (2008) Effectiveness of tai chi for Parkinson's disease: A critical review. *Parkinsonism & Related Disorders*, 14(8): 589–594

Lücking, C.B., Dürr, A., Bonifati, V., Vaughan, J., De Michele, G., Gasser, T., Harhangi, B.S., Meco, G., Denefle, P., Wood, N.W., Agid, Y. & Brice, A. (2000) Association between early onset Parkinson's disease and mutations in the parkin gene. *New England Journal of Medicine*, 342: 1560–1567

National Collaborating Centre for Chronic Conditions (2006) *Parkinson's disease: National clinical guidelines for diagnosis and management in primary and secondary care.* London: Royal College of Physicians

National Collaborating Centre for Mental Health (2007) *Dementia: Supporting individuals with dementia and their carers in health and social care.* NICE clinical guideline 42. Leicester and London: The British Psychological Society and the Royal College of Psychiatrists

Valente, E.M., Abou-Sleiman, P.M., Caputo, V., Muqit, M.M., Harvey, K., Gispert, S., Ali, Z., Del Turco, D., Bentivoglio, A.R., Healy, D.G., Albanese, A., Nussbaum, R., Gonzalez-Maldonado, R., Deller, T., Salvi, S., Cortelli, P., Gilks, W.P., Latchman, D.S., Harvey, R.J., Dallapiccola, B., Auburger, G. & Wood, N.W. (2004) Hereditary early onset Parkinson's disease caused by mutations in PINK1. *Science*, 304: 1158–1160

USEFUL WEBSITES

Brain & Spine Foundation – www.brainandspine.org.uk

Howard Hughes Medical Institute – www.hhmi.org

National Collaborating Centre for Chronic Conditions – www.rcplondon.ac.uk

National Collaborating Centre for Mental Health – www.rcplondon.ac.uk

National Institute for Health and Clinical Excellence – www.nice.org.uk

Parkinson's UK – www.parkinsons.org.uk

MULTIPLE SCLEROSIS

KEYPOINTS

- Multiple sclerosis (MS) is a chronic, progressive, degenerative long-term disorder that affects nerve fibres in the brain and in the spinal cord.
- MS slows down nerve impulses and can result in weakness, numbness, pain and loss of vision.
- Most individuals with MS have a relatively normal lifespan and life expectancy is about 35 years after onset of the condition.
- After 25 years or so, approximately two-thirds of those with MS are able to remain mobile. The disorder eventually results in physical limitations in about 70% of sufferers.
- An estimated 2.5 million individuals in the world are thought to have MS.
- Generally across the globe, the prevalence increases the further away you travel from the equator.
- MS is diagnosed in about 1820 to 3380 new individuals each year in England and Wales.
- It is estimated that in England there is a mean total cost per patient of £17,000 per year, suggesting a total burden to society of around £1.34 billion per year.
- The main focus of any physical activity programme would normally be to improve the capability of the individual with MS to perform activities of daily living as this disease can be extremely debilitating.
- Even though limited research has been carried out on the effects of physical activity on MS sufferers, some reported benefits include the following:
  - improved health and well-being
  - ability to maintain or improve function
  - a reduction in the impact of relapses
  - reduced muscle loss and maintenance of strength
  - improved postural control
  - reduced spasticity occurrence.

WHAT IS IT?

Multiple sclerosis (MS) can be classed as a chronic, progressive, degenerative disorder that affects nerve fibres (called axons) in the brain and in the spinal cord (in combination known as the central nervous system). In simple terms, this means that multiple sclerosis is considered to be a long-term disorder that gets worse over time although, fortunately, most individuals who have the disease go on to have a normal lifespan. It is generally known that the disease is caused when the fatty substance that surrounds and insulates nerve fibres (called myelin sheaths) becomes damaged in certain places, which subsequently affects the transmission of nerve impulses (electrical signals that pass along nerves) at the damaged areas. Multiple sclerosis is also known as an 'autoimmune disease', as damage to the nerve fibre myelin insulation is usually caused by the individual's own immune system. This damage to the myelin insulation is more technically known as 'demyelination' and is caused by the destruction of specialised cells (which are called oligodendrocytes)

that form the fatty myelin substance. As a result of this demyelination, scarring and hardening of nerve fibres can occur in either the spinal cord, brain stem or optic nerves. This has the effect of slowing down nerve impulses and can lead to weakness, numbness, pain and loss of vision. The scarring and hardening of the nerves is known as 'sclerosis', which is where the disease gets its name from: multiple areas of scarring. In individuals who have this particular disease, symptoms can either get worse (exacerbation) or improve, and can also develop in different areas of the body at different times. Depending on the nature of the symptoms presented, multiple sclerosis can be classified as one of four types (although not all sources agree on this), as shown in table 11.1.

One of the main reasons for having the different classifications of multiple sclerosis is that the history of the disease, as identified by the particular subtype, can help to predict the future course of the disease, which in turn can help the specialist with decisions relating to specific treatment and therapy. The majority of individuals who have been diagnosed with the disease have a

Table 11.1	Classifications of MS
Type	**Description**
Primary progressive MS	Steady progression of symptoms with few periods of remission
Relapsing-remitting MS (about 80% have this type at onset)	Unpredictable worsening of symptoms (exacerbations) that occur with increasing frequency, along with periods of reduced symptoms (remission)
Secondary progressive MS (also called 'galloping MS')	Similar to relapsing-remitting MS; eventually progresses to MS with no remission
Progressive-relapsing MS	Accumulative damage during exacerbations and remissions, and suffer a steady decline; this is the least common of the subtypes

relatively normal lifespan and life expectancy. Generally speaking, this is about 35 years after onset of the disease. Research also shows that, after about 25 years or so, approximately two-thirds of all those with MS are able to remain mobile and carry out their normal daily functions. It should be pointed out, however, that the disease does eventually result in certain physical limitations in about 70% of all sufferers. With regard to the history of the disease, even though clinical details had been described in the early 1800s, a French neurologist by the name of Jean-Martin Charcot (1825–1893) was the first individual to recognise multiple sclerosis as a separate disease in 1868. At the time Charcot called the disease 'sclerose en plaques' before it was later renamed to become what is now known as multiple sclerosis. It is also interesting to note that in the early research by Charcot he referred to cognition changes, describing his patients as having an 'enfeeblement of the memory' and 'conceptions that formed slowly', which are symptoms that are now commonly associated with multiple sclerosis.

PREVALENCE

According to the National Collaboration Centre for Chronic Conditions, an estimated 2.5 million individuals in the world are thought to have one of the classifications of multiple sclerosis. Generally across the globe, the prevalence increases the further away from the equator you travel, as decreased sunlight has been linked with a higher risk of the disease. For example, those parts of Asia, Africa and America that lie on the equator have extremely low levels of the disease, while places

such as Canada and Scotland, which lie far from the equator, have particularly high rates of the disease. In relation to statistics for the UK there is as yet no national register for those with multiple sclerosis, however according to the Multiple Sclerosis Trust, it is estimated that about 1820 to 3380 new cases of multiple sclerosis are diagnosed each year in England and Wales, where it is usually diagnosed in individuals between the ages of 20 and 50. The trust also estimates the total number of cases in the UK to be between 85,000 and 100,000. Strangely, once multiple sclerosis has been diagnosed, individuals often realise that they have had the disease for many years but just didn't identify the symptoms. In terms of gender difference, it is estimated that multiple sclerosis affects two women for each man among those who are affected. Although the total number of those with MS may be small in comparison to certain other conditions, the disease still has quite a considerable cost element. For example, it has been estimated that, in England alone, there is a mean total cost per patient of £17,000 per year, suggesting a total burden to society of around £1.34 billion per year, of which most of the cost is borne by the NHS.

RISK FACTORS

It is widely thought that the average age at which individuals develop multiple sclerosis seems to be between the age of 18 and 35, however the disease has been known to develop at any age (both younger and older). In terms of the wide range of research that has been done in relation to the disease, there are many credible sources which suggest that children of parents with multiple sclerosis have a higher rate of incidence (30–50% higher). It should be pointed out, though, that there are many other sources which argue that multiple sclerosis is not a hereditary disease, even though there are a number of genetic variations that have been suggested to increase the risk of developing the disease. As well as the potential genetic link, exposure to a virus such as the common cold, influenza or gastroenteritis has also been suggested to trigger the disease. A specific viral risk factor has not yet been identified, but exposure to a virus that causes demyelination (especially prior to adolescence) may be a risk factor. Even though the specific cause of multiple sclerosis is not yet fully understood and there is still debate regarding the genetic link, the higher incidence of the disease in certain geographical areas and the fact that relapses occur more frequently during spring and summer leads scientists to believe that environmental factors may be involved. There are also several other factors that have been suggested to be linked to the disease. For example, it is thought that certain mechanisms of stress may trigger an attack as can the condition of pregnancy. It appears that, in the case of pregnancy, research shows that during the first few months after the delivery of the baby, the risk of relapse is increased. Overall, though, research also shows that pregnancy does not seem to influence long-term disability. With this particular disease, most risk factors are non-modifiable, except perhaps for reducing or dealing with the effects of stress.

SYMPTOMS

When an individual develops multiple sclerosis, early symptoms may appear, which may be brief and mild. Symptoms such as vision changes (e.g.

blurred vision, blind spots) and muscle weakness can present themselves and progress steadily over time. Symptoms can also occur as acute attacks or flare-ups (also called exacerbations) followed by a partial or complete reduction in symptoms (known as remission). Periods of relapse are often unpredictable and can occur without warning, however they rarely occur at a frequency of more than twice per year. There are many potential symptoms of multiple sclerosis, which include those in table 11.2, but it is important to note that individuals with the disease can suffer from any of them at any time.

DIAGNOSIS

Multiple sclerosis can be a difficult disease to diagnose accurately as the signs and symptoms can be similar to those related to other medical problems. As cost can be an issue in relation to diagnostic equipment and expertise, different diagnostic methods have been explored. For instance, there have been many medical organisations that have designed specific diagnostic criteria tools that have tried to address the cost implication, such as the McDonald criteria and the Expanded Disability Status Score (EDSS). However, although costly, one of the most commonly used diagnostic tools is that of neuroimaging, in which images of the brain are examined using methods such as magnetic resonance imaging (MRI), which can highlight areas of demyelination. Another diagnostic method that is often used is the analysis of cerebrospinal fluid obtained from a lumbar puncture in which chemical signs of inflammation can be used to detect the disease. A less common

Table 11.2	Common symptoms of MS
Symptom	**Description**
Ataxia	This is the term given to balance problems such as dizziness, vertigo, uncoordinated movements and tremor
Hypoesthesia and paraesthesia	This refers to changes in sensation
Dysarthria	This is another term for general speech problems
Dysphagia	This relates to difficulty in swallowing, which is a quite common symptom of the disease
Nystagmus, optic neuritis or diplopia	These terms all relate to vision abnormalities such as eye pain, vision loss in one eye, double vision and involuntary eye movement
Lhermitte's sign	This refers to an electrical sensation that runs down the back when bending the neck
Cognitive dysfunction	Multiple sclerosis can lead to a range of cognitive effects, such as poor memory, poor reasoning or difficulty in maintaining concentration
Behavioural dysfunction	This can refer to any condition such as anxiety, mood swings and depression
Bladder and bowel dysfunction	This relates to any dysfunction such as urgency, incontinence or constipation
Motor abnormalities	This relates to muscle weakness, spasticity (rigid muscles) or muscle spasm
Fatigue	Because of the mental and physical problems associated with multiple sclerosis, fitness can suffer as a result, which often leads to fatigue

method is the use of small electrical currents (known as evoked potentials), which are sometimes used to try to stimulate the optic nerve and sensory nerves. This is done because the nervous system of an individual with multiple sclerosis responds less actively to stimulation due to demyelination of the pathways. According to the National Collaboration Centre for Chronic Conditions, there are specific issues relating to the diagnosis of multiple sclerosis that highlight the difficulty with diagnosis. The specific issues include those listed below.

- Individuals may have or may develop one or more of a large range of specific problems.
- Individuals may have problems that are not always obvious and even the individual with multiple sclerosis may be unaware of them.
- Individuals may be unaware that something can be done to alleviate problems and so may not mention them.
- Individuals may be in touch with someone who focuses on only one problem, and who may fail to detect or know about others, consequently not referring the individual on to appropriate services for further treatment.

PHYSICAL ACTIVITY BENEFITS

Many of the published benefits of physical activity relate to a reduction of the symptoms of the disease rather than as a rehabilitation tool for the condition. For instance, regular physical activity can help to increase cardiovascular fitness and muscular strength, which is often lost as a result of developing multiple sclerosis. Unfortunately, only limited research has been carried out on the effects of physical activity on multiple sclerosis sufferers,

however in 2003 the National Institute for Health and Clinical Excellence (NICE) reported that the benefits of physical activity included the following:

- improved health and well-being
- ability to maintain or improve function
- a reduction in the impact of relapses
- reduced muscle loss and maintenance of strength
- improved postural control
- reduced spasticity occurrence.

Table 11.3	Physical activity guidelines for individuals with multiple sclerosis	
	Aerobic training	**Strength training**
Mode	• Large-muscle activities (e.g. walking, cycling, swimming)	• Isokinetic machines, weight machines, free weights; train one side of the body then the other (unilateral)
Intensity	• 60–85% of HRmax • 10–15 RPE	• Use loads up to 50% of maximum • Overload by increasing repetitions then intensity
Duration	• 20–30 minutes per session • Increase the duration rather than intensity • Slow progression taking account of relapses	• Perform 2 to 3 sets of 12–15 RM • 1–2 minutes' rest between exercises
Frequency	• 3 sessions per week	• 2–3 sessions per week • Encourage other forms of exercise • Reduce in periods of relapse
Precautions	• Use shorter sessions if needed, to avoid fatigue • Do not do activities during a relapse • Avoid high impact for those with foot problems	• Avoid muscular fatigue • Balance upper and lower body • Do on non-aerobic days

General precautions
- See table 11.4

PHYSICAL ACTIVITY GUIDELINES

With this particular disease, people wishing to supervise activities for those with multiple sclerosis would only be able to do so following close liaison with a qualified individual, however an understanding of guidelines relating to physical activity is still useful. The main focus of any physical activity programme would normally be to improve the capability of the individual with MS to perform activities of daily living as this disease can be extremely debilitating. Most individuals with the disease would have relatively low aerobic capacity levels, therefore short sessions of low intensity would be recommended as a starting point for any programme. The other main point for supervisors to remember is that those with MS often have poor balance as a result of the disease, so programmes should take this into account in terms of safety and for prescription purposes. Table 11.3 gives an overview of the physical activity guidelines related to individuals with MS.

Due to the complex nature of this particular disease and the debilitating effects that it can have, there are several precautions (see the examples in table 11.4) that should be taken when working with those who have been diagnosed with multiple sclerosis, regardless of the type (or classification) as described in table 11.1. However, as mentioned before, supervisors should seek advice when working with individuals who have MS.

Table 11.4	Physical activity precautions for MS
Precaution	**Comment**
Start off with short intermittent cardio sessions	Fatigue can reduce physical activity tolerance
Always stay close to the client during all exercises and avoid any activities that challenge balance too much	MS sufferers usually have impaired balance and coordination
Wear appropriate clothing and take water breaks often	MS sufferers usually have impaired heat tolerance and can dehydrate easily
Discuss foot problems with the client	Spasticity may lead to requirement for foot strapping or braces of some nature
Discuss individual, domestic and social issues with the individual so that goals can be set	Individual activities such as dressing, eating and washing; domestic activities such as cooking, washing, ironing and cleaning; social activities such as shopping, clubs, etc.

RECOMMENDED READING

American College of Sports Medicine (2009a) *ACSM's exercise management for persons with chronic diseases and disabilities* (3rd edn). Champaign, IL: Human Kinetics

American College of Sports Medicine (2009b) *ACSM's guidelines for exercise testing and prescription* (8th edn). London: Lippincott Williams & Wilkins

Ascherio, A. & Munger, K.L. (2007) Environmental risk factors for multiple sclerosis. Part I: The role of infection. *Annals of Neurology*, 61(4): 288–299

Compston, A. & Coles, A. (2008) Multiple sclerosis. *Lancet*, 372(9648): 1502–1517

Compston, A., Ebers, G., Lassmann, H., McDonald, J., Matthews, P.M. & Wekerle, H. (1998) *McAlpine's multiple sclerosis* (3rd edn). London: Churchill Livingstone

Dyment, D.A., Ebers, G.C. & Sadovnick, A.D. (2004) Genetics of multiple sclerosis. *Lancet Neurology*, 3(2): 104–110

Gronseth, G.S. & Ashman, E.J. (2000) Practice parameter: The usefulness of evoked potentials in identifying clinically silent lesions in patients with suspected multiple sclerosis (an evidence-based review): Report of the Quality Standards Subcommittee of the American Academy of Neurology. *Neurology*, 54(9): 1720–1725

Heesen, C., Mohr, D.C., Huitinga, I., Bergh, F.T., Gaab, J., Otte, C. & Gold, S.M. (2007) Stress regulation in multiple sclerosis: Current issues and concepts. *Multiple Sclerosis*, 13(2): 143–148

Khan, F., Turner-Stokes, L., Ng, L. & Kilpatrick, T. (2007) Multidisciplinary rehabilitation for adults with multiple sclerosis. *Cochrane Database of Systematic Reviews*, 2: CD 006036

Kurtzke, J.F. (1983) Rating neurologic impairment in multiple sclerosis: An expanded disability status scale (EDSS). *Neurology*, 33(11): 1444–1452

Marrie, R.A. (2004) Environmental risk factors in multiple sclerosis aetiology. *Lancet Neurology*, 3(12): 709–718

McDonald, W.I., Compston, A., Edan, G., Goodkin, D., Hartung, H.P., Lublin, F.D., McFarland, H.F., Paty, D.W., Polman, C.H., Reingold, S.C., Sandberg-Wollheim, M., Sibley, W., Thompson, A., van den Noort, S., Weinshenker, B.Y. & Wolinsky, J.S. (2001) Recommended diagnostic criteria for multiple sclerosis: Guidelines from the International Panel on the diagnosis of multiple sclerosis. *Annals of Neurology*, 50(1): 121–127

Miller, D., Barkhof, F., Montalban, X., Thompson, A. & Filippi, M. (2005) Clinically isolated syndromes suggestive of multiple sclerosis, part I: Natural history, pathogenesis, diagnosis, and prognosis. *Lancet Neurology*, 4(5): 281–288

Miller, D.H. & Leary, S.M. (2007) Primary-progressive multiple sclerosis. *Lancet Neurology*, 6(10): 903–912

National Collaborating Centre for Chronic Conditions (2004) *Multiple sclerosis. National clinical guideline for diagnosis and management in primary and secondary care.* London: Royal College of Physicians

National Institute for Health and Clinical Excellence (NICE) (2003) *Multiple sclerosis: Management of multiple sclerosis in primary and secondary care.* Clinical Guideline 8. London: NICE

Pearce, J.M. (2005) Historical descriptions of multiple sclerosis. *European Neurology*, 54(1): 49–53

Poser, C.M. & Brinar, V.V. (2004) Diagnostic criteria for multiple sclerosis: An historical review. *Clinical Neurology and Neurosurgery*, 106(3): 147–158

Rashid, W. & Miller, D.H. (2008) Recent advances in neuroimaging of multiple sclerosis. *Seminars in Neurology*, 28(1): 46–55

Rosati, G. (2001) The prevalence of multiple sclerosis in the world: An update. *Neurological Sciences*, 22: 117–139

Rovaris, M., Confavreux, C., Furlan, R., Kappos, L., Comi, G. & Filippi, M. (2006) Secondary progressive multiple sclerosis: Current knowledge and future challenges. *Lancet Neurology*, 5(4): 343–354

Tataru, N., Vidal, C., Decavel, P., Berger, E. & Rumbach, L. (2006) Limited impact of the summer heat wave in France (2003) on hospital admissions and relapses for multiple sclerosis. *Neuroepidemiology*, 27(1): 28–32

Trojano, M. & Paolicelli, D. (2001) The differential diagnosis of multiple sclerosis: Classification and clinical features of relapsing and progressive neurological syndromes. *Neurological Sciences*, 22(suppl. 2): S98–S102

Weinshenker, B.G. (1994) Natural history of multiple sclerosis. *Annals of Neurology*, 36 (Suppl): S6–S11

USEFUL WEBSITES

American Academy of Neurology – www.aan.com

Cochrane Collaboration (Cochrane Reviews) – www.cochrane.org

Multiple Sclerosis Society – www.mssociety.org.uk

Multiple Sclerosis Trust – www.mstrust.org.uk

National Collaborating Centre for Chronic Conditions – www.rcplondon.ac.uk

National Institute for Health and Clinical Excellence – www.nice.org

CARDIO-VASCULAR DISEASE (CVD)

12

KEYPOINTS

- Cardiovascular disease (CVD) affects 13.6% of men and 13% of women in the UK each year, causing 216,000 deaths.
- Coronary heart disease (CHD) is recognised as the biggest killer in the country, responsible for killing more than 110,000 individuals in England alone every year.
- It is estimated that more than 1.4 million individuals suffer from angina and 275,000 individuals have a heart attack annually.
- Physical activity can help prevent CHD in men and women. Inactive and unfit individuals have almost double the risk of dying from CHD compared with more active and fit individuals.
- Physical activity also significantly reduces the risk of stroke and provides effective treatment of peripheral vascular disease.
- Physical activity helps to improve several risk factors for CVD, including raised blood pressure, adverse blood lipids and insulin resistance.
- Thirty minutes of at least moderate-intensity physical activity a day on at least five days a week can reduce the risk of CVD.
- Shorter bouts of physical activity, of 10 minutes or more, interspersed throughout the day can be as effective as longer sessions of activity (as long as the total energy expended is the same).
- Exercise-based rehabilitation programmes for patients with CHD are generally effective in reducing cardiac deaths and may also be effective in the rehabilitation of individuals with stroke.
- For individuals with peripheral vascular disease exercise (PVD) rehabilitation can improve walking ability and the ability to perform everyday tasks.

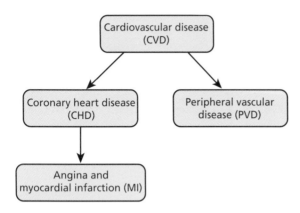

Figure 12.1 Common terms related to heart disease

WHAT IS IT?

There are many terms that are used, often incorrectly, when referring to any particular form of heart disease. Fig 12.1 shows how the most commonly used terms relate to one another.

Even though there are slight differences between the terms, they are often used interchangeably by individuals to mean the same thing. Cardiovascular disease (CVD) is the umbrella term for a range of conditions that can affect the heart and the network of veins and arteries that transport blood around the body. Any type of CVD can have detrimental effects on an individual's quality of life. One of the CVD types is that of coronary heart disease (CHD), which is classed as a preventable disease of which there are two subcategories known as 'angina' and 'myocardial infarction' (MI). The other type of CVD is peripheral vascular disease (PVD), which relates to blockage of the arteries.

ANGINA

The correct term for this subcategory of CHD is 'angina pectoris' (derived loosely from the Greek meaning 'strangling chest') and is commonly associated with severe chest pain as it describes symptoms rather than being an actual disease. Angina occurs as a result of a build-up of deposits on the artery walls (known as atherosclerosis), which results in the flow of blood through the narrowed vessel being restricted. If this occurs, the amount of oxygen to tissues being fed by the blocked arteries is reduced (see fig 7.3 on page 96). Angina can be classified as either 'stable' or 'unstable' depending on the presentation of the condition. If symptoms occur as a result of an increase in activity, and have a predictable pattern, then it is referred to as 'stable angina'. If symptoms occur for no particular reason then it is referred to as 'unstable angina'.

MYOCARDIAL INFARCTION (MI)

Due to the atherosclerosis build-up of lipids (fats) and fibrous tissue within the coronary arteries (arteries that supply the heart), blood can be prevented or restricted from flowing through them. As a result, this would reduce the transportation of oxygen to the heart. When this happens it is generally known as 'ischemia', but in the case of the heart it is known as 'coronary ischemia'. If this situation is prolonged it can cause death of the cells leading to a myocardial infarction (MI), which is more commonly known as a heart attack. This normally affects the ability of the left ventricle (which is the chamber within the heart that pumps blood out through the arteries) to contract and deliver oxygen to the body.

PERIPHERAL VASCULAR DISEASE (PVD)

The other type of cardiovascular disease is known as peripheral vascular disease (PVD), which is also known sometimes as peripheral artery disease (PAD) or peripheral artery occlusive disease (PAOD). This particular disease is mainly related to atherosclerosis of the peripheral arteries (any arteries other than those around the heart or brain), which is when fatty deposits are stored on the inside of the arteries, resulting in a thickening of the arterial walls and a narrowing of the lumen (this is the space in the artery through which the blood flows). As atherosclerosis develops it causes a restriction of blood flow, which is most common in the lower extremities, particularly affecting the legs and ankles (this may be only on one side). PVD can also be caused as a result of an embolism or thrombus (blood clots that become lodged in the arteries). The disease creates great difficulty with regards to the ability an individual has to walk and can cause severe pain, especially when doing any form of physical exertion.

PREVALENCE

In 2003, the World Health Organization (WHO) stated that CVD was responsible for 29% of global deaths every year, putting the figure at around 16.7 million individuals. Also, according to the Department of Epidemiology and Public Health in the same year, CVD affected 13.6% of the men and 13% of women in the UK, causing 216,000 deaths and creating a total cost to the UK of £17.38 billion. As far as CHD is concerned, it is recognised as the biggest killer in the country, responsible for killing more than 110,000 individuals in England alone every year. It is also estimated that more than 1.4 million individuals have angina and 275,000 individuals have a heart attack annually. According to the Department of Health, the government was committed to reducing the death rate from CHD and stroke and related diseases in individuals under the age of 75 by at least 40% (to 83.8 deaths per 100,000 population) by 2010. As far as peripheral vascular disease is concerned, even though the disease is not considered to be life threatening, the levels of associated pain can be very severe. The prevalence of PVD increases with age. According to Fowkes *et al.* (1991), about 3% of people under the age of 60 have the disease, but this rises to over 20% in people over the age of 75 years. Fowkes also states that only a quarter of those affected by PVD have symptoms, and it is more common in men than women.

SYMPTOMS

ANGINA

Individuals with angina commonly suffer symptoms such as shortness of breath, nausea, sweating, and pain across the front of the chest, which can radiate to the shoulders, arms, neck and jaw. It is often described as a crushing or strangling feeling on the chest. This generally lasts for a few seconds but can continue for as long as 30 minutes.

MYOCARDIAL INFARCTION

Symptoms of a myocardial infarction (MI) usually occur gradually over a few minutes rather than as a sudden onset. Chest pain that radiates to the left arm and sometimes to the lower jaw, neck, right arm and back is the most common symptom.

Sufferers can also experience shortness of breath (known as dyspnoea) because the damage to the heart as a result of the MI reduces the ability for oxygen to be transported to the muscles. There is also a tendency to sweat excessively, with heart palpitations, which can result in the sufferer feeling light-headed and nauseous. Interestingly, about half of all MI patients have stated that they have experienced symptoms such as chest pain prior to the infarction and, in some cases, up to a month before the event. It is important to know that the early phases of myocardial infarction and acute angina can be very similar. It is also worth noting that approximately a quarter of all myocardial infarctions have been known to occur with no symptoms whatsoever.

PERIPHERAL VASCULAR DISEASE

As peripheral vascular disease (PVD) is related to decreased blood flow, sufferers often experience pain (known as claudication), weakness, numbness and cramping in the muscles. Sores, wounds and ulcers can also appear, which heal slowly or sometimes do not heal at all. A limb affected by

Table 12.1	Cardiovascular disease (CVD) symptoms
Dyspnoea	Shortness of breath occurs in everyday life but can also suggest early signs of CVD. It can be categorised into three basic types: pulmonary, functional and cardiac. Pulmonary dyspnoea affects oxygen transport to the lungs. Functional dyspnoea is related to psychological areas such as anxiety, and can lead to hyperventilation. Cardiac dyspnoea is brought on by obstructions within the arteries or by a weakening of the heart muscle.
Chest pain	When oxygen to the heart is restricted, a 'squeezing' pain is felt in the chest, which can also radiate to the shoulder and down the left arm. If the pain goes away it suggests angina, but if it does not go away after a period of rest, it suggests a heart attack.
Palpitations	This is when the heart beats very rapidly (known as arrhythmia), which can occur without any physical exertion at all. It can continue for several minutes and is known as an indication of CVD.
Syncope	Syncope (fainting) occurs when the brain is starved of oxygenated blood for more than a few seconds. This can be caused by a slow heart beat, low blood pressure, blocked blood vessels or a narrowing of a heart valve.
Oedema	This is when lymph fluid or water is retained within cells and causes swellings. Common areas of swelling include legs, eyes, ankles, abdominal and chest walls. Swelling can also occur when the muscle on the right side of the heart is weak, causing a build-up of pressure and resulting in oedema in the legs and abdomen.
Cyanosis	This refers to a lack of oxygenated blood flowing through capillaries, causing a blue-like discoloration of the skin (mainly around the lips and fingernails).
Claudication	This is the primary symptom of PVD and is often described as walking-induced pain in one or both legs, which does not go away with continued walking and is relieved by rest. It mainly affects the calves but can also affect the buttocks and radiate down the legs.

PVD can also seem paler (or even blue) and colder when compared to the other normal limb. Claudication affects up to 40% of all those with PVD and this can drastically affect their fitness and daily activity levels by as much as 50%, and many to such an extent that they become housebound and immobile. In severe cases of the disease this can lead to amputation of the affected limb.

Some of the symptoms of all three conditions are similar and often have clinical names associated with them. Table 12.1 gives an overview and description of the more common cardiovascular disease symptoms.

RISK FACTORS

According to the NHS Information Centre, obese men are more likely to have CVD than those who are of a normal weight (17% compared with 10%) and obese women are more likely to have CVD than women of normal weight (15% compared with 9%). The Centre also stated that both men and women with a raised waist circumference were more likely to have CVD than those without a raised waist circumference. Even though there are common risk factors associated with CVD, there are specific ones related to each subcategory, as can be seen in tables 12.2, 12.3 and 12.4. As with risk factors related to other diseases, some of the CVD risk factors are classed as modifiable and others are classed as non-modifiable.

DIAGNOSIS

As testing for angina, MI and PVD is vastly different in terms of the diagnosis and the tests used, each one will be considered in turn.

Table 12.2	Risk factors for angina, MI and PVD
Risk factor	**Description**
Age	Risk increases with age, especially ≥55 yrs for men and ≥65 yrs for women
Smoking	The risk increases with the amount (this is not a linear increase though)
Diabetes mellitus (DM)	The risk is increased with diabetes
Dyslipidaemia	The risk is increased if cholesterol levels are high
Family history of premature CVD	There is a genetic link for family history in males <55 yrs and females <65yrs
Hypertension	Elevated blood pressure is linked with an increase in the risk of developing PVD
Obesity	For those with a BMI ≥30 kg/m^2 the risk is increased
Sedentary	Sedentary behaviour can greatly increase the risk of angina

Table 12.3	Risk factors for myocardial infarction (MI)
Risk factor	**Description**
Diabetes	Considered one of the most important risk factors for ischemic heart disease (IHD)
Smoking	The risk increases with the amount (this is not a linear increase, though)
Hypercholesterolemia	Certain levels of cholesterol can affect risk (high levels of low-density lipoprotein and low levels of high-density lipoprotein)
Hypertension	Elevated blood pressure is linked with an increase in the risk of developing PVD
Family history of ischemic heart disease (IHD)	Risk is increased if there is a family history
Obesity	For those with a BMI $\geq$30 kg/m^2 the risk is increased
Age	Risk is increased for men at age 45 and women at age 55
Hyperhomocysteinaemia	High blood levels of homocysteine (a toxic amino acid) that is elevated when intakes of vitamins B$_2$, B$_6$, B$_{12}$ and folic acid are low
Alcohol	Studies show that prolonged exposure to high quantities of alcohol can increase the risk of heart attack
Gender	Males are more at risk than females
Sedentary	Individuals who are active are 1.9 times less likely to have a heart attack than inactive individuals

Table 12.4	Risk factors for peripheral vascular disease PVD
Risk factor	**Description**
Smoking	Smokers have up to a tenfold increase in relative risk for PVD
Diabetes	There is between a two and four times increased risk of PVD for diabetics; a diabetic who smokes runs an approximately 30% risk of amputation within five years
Dyslipidaemia	Elevation of total cholesterol, LDL-cholesterol and triglyceride levels each have been linked to accelerated PVD
Hypertension	Elevated blood pressure is linked with an increase in the risk of developing PVD
Age	Risk of PVD increases over the age of 50
Obesity	For those with a BMI $\geq$30 kg/m^2 the risk is increased

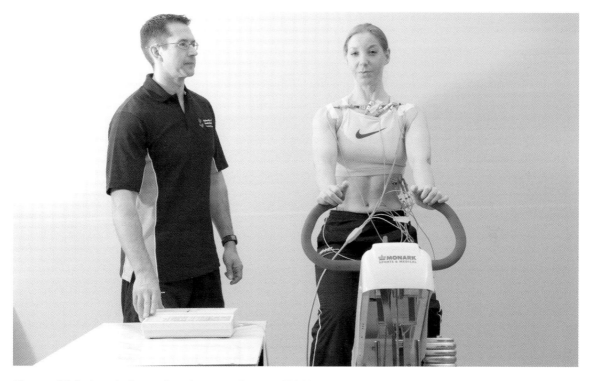

Figure 12.2 A typical exercise electrocardiogram (ECG) test

TESTING FOR ANGINA

Due to the severe nature of this condition, only clinical testing by suitably qualified individuals is carried out. Normally an exercise electrocardiogram test (see fig 12.2) is performed (known as an ECG test, which is a treadmill test done while monitoring the heart). In this particular test, the patient exercises to their maximum ability before fatigue, breathlessness or pain occurs. The results of the ECG test, known as a monitor trace, are then analysed by a qualified individual in order to help form a diagnosis of angina. There are other alternatives to an ECG exercise test for those who are not able to exercise to a sufficiently high level. For instance an 'angiography' imaging test can also be done. This is where a fine, flexible tube, known as a catheter, is inserted into the artery of the patient (often the femoral artery in the groin area) and guided to the suspected blocked vessel where a dye is injected through the catheter into the artery. An X-ray is then taken immediately, which should be able to identify any blockage.

TESTING FOR MI

For obvious reasons, the diagnosis of a MI can be made only following the actual event. If the person who had the event is fortunate enough to survive, then a physical examination using a combination of an electrocardiogram and blood tests is normally carried out in a clinical environment. The purpose of this is to look for evidence of any damage to the heart muscle. If symptoms have resolved themselves by the time of the evaluation, further tests can then be carried out to investigate if there are any areas of reduced blood flow that might have resulted from or even caused the infarction.

TESTING FOR PVD

If PVD is suspected, a measure of the fall in blood pressure in the arteries supplying the legs is usually carried out, again in a clinical environment. The standard test that is done is known as the 'ankle brachial pressure index' (ABPI) test, which measures the difference between arm blood pressure and ankle blood pressure. If the test result identifies a problem, a lower-limb Doppler ultrasound examination is then normally done, which can provide a real-time image of the arteries (in particular the suspected site) and also the extent of any artery blockage. Angiography and computerised tomography (CT) scanning are alternative methods that can be used.

PHYSICAL ACTIVITY BENEFITS

There are many published sources relating to the benefits of physical activity for CVD. Table 12.5 gives an overview of the more common benefits

that have been taken from a variety of those published sources.

In terms of research, there are many studies that support the prescription of 30 minutes per day of moderate-intensity activity in order to reduce the risk of CVD. For example, in a study known as the Women's Health Initiative, nearly 74,000 post-menopausal women aged 50 to 79 years participated, which required them to walk briskly for at least 2.5 hours per week. The study resulted in a 30% reduction in cardiovascular events over three years of follow-up. Also in the Nurses' Health Study, 72,000 healthy middle-aged female nurses who walked briskly for three hours per week were followed for eight years and found to have a 30–40% lower incidence of heart attack compared to sedentary women (both studies led by Manson; see Manson *et al.*, 1999, 2002). Similar findings have also been reported with men as the subjects. For instance, in the Health Professionals Follow-up Study by Tanasescu and colleagues (2002), a 12-year follow-up of 44,000 healthy male health professionals aged 40 to 75 years who did ahalf-hour per day or more of brisk walking found an 18% reduction in heart disease incidence. Also, in general, there are many studies related to men which suggest that vigorous

Table 12.5	Typical benefits of physical activity for CVD	
Angina	**Myocardial infarction**	**Peripheral vascular disease**
• Lower blood pressure • Lower heart response to submaximal exertion • Lower heart muscle O_2 demands • Improved functional capacity • Relief of angina symptoms	• Increased aerobic capacity (VO_2) • Reduced heart rate, blood cholesterol and blood pressure • Improved well-being	• Improved pain response • Improved gait • Improved quality of life

physical activity is associated with even greater reductions in the risk of CVD than is moderate-intensity activity. Studies such as that by Selig and Hare (2006) have also looked at those individuals with 'chronic heart failure' (CHF), and shown that combinations of moderate aerobic and strength training programmes can improve aerobic capacity, muscular function and peripheral blood flow.

PHYSICAL ACTIVITY GUIDELINES

It is important to note that individuals in this particular population will either be under direct physician supervision or have specific prescribed physical activity guidelines following appropriate testing, and will be referred to a particular centre for supervision of a physical activity programme. Those who are supervising individuals from this population should be suitably qualified (minimum British Association of Cardiac Rehabilitation (BACR) phase IV), therefore it is their role to facilitate the prescribed physical activity programme and be fully aware of the respective condition for supervisory purposes. The supervisor should also be fully aware that if individuals display certain conditions at any time (known as contraindications) then any further physical activity should not be undertaken, and this information should be relayed directly to the relevant physician. Contraindications for those with any form of CVD should have been identified in a clinical environment, but if a supervisor should become aware of any contraindications that have not previously been identified then they should refer the individual back to the specialist for further consultation. The contraindications that a supervisor should look out for are the following:

- unstable angina
- either systolic blood pressure equal to or above 180 mmHg or diastolic equal to or above 100 mmHg
- resting heart rate above 100 bpm
- uncontrolled atrial or ventricular arrhythmias (abnormal heart beat)
- unstable or acute heart failure
- unstable diabetes
- febrile illness (fever-like).

Those individuals who supervise activities for cardiac patients should know that in some cases when the restriction of blood flow through the arteries is quite severe and other ways of trying to increase the blood flow do not work, an artery bypass operation may be carried out (this is known as a coronary artery bypass graft, or CABG), in order to bypass the affected vessels. If this is not done then the affected vessel may be widened by inserting a metal cage known as a stent. This operation is called an 'angioplasty'. When these operations are successful, the blood flow and oxygen supply is increased, which helps to reduce (or in some cases eliminate) the symptoms of angina or ischemia. Care must be taken, however, to ensure that any individual who has been through either of these procedures has enough time to fully recover before undertaking any physical activity programme. In relation to guidelines for physical activity, even though there are similarities between the three main areas of CVD it is best to separate each main area (angina, MI and PVD).

Table 12.6	Physical activity guidelines for individuals who have angina	
	Aerobic training	**Strength training**
Mode	• Walking, cycling and water-based activity, as for any other condition • Individuals normally undergo a progression of initial, improvement and maintenance phases	• Use a combination of free weights and body weight • Use functional exercises such as standing to sitting squats or lifting tins on and off a shelf • Include mobility of the thoracic spine
Intensity	• Prolonged warm-up and cool-down • Encourage the individual to exercise about 10–20 beats below the angina threshold	• Use loads up to 40–50% of maximum voluntary contraction • Overload by increasing repetitions then intensity • Increase intensity by 5% when ready
Duration	• 5–10 minutes per session • Short bouts with rest periods are advised • Increase duration rather than intensity	• Perform 3 sets of 10–15 RM • 1–2 minutes' rest between exercises • 8–10 exercises
Frequency	• 1–2 times a day • 4–6 days per week	• 2–3 sessions per week
Precaution	• Exercising in the cold can trigger the symptoms • Water-based activities can be hazardous • Avoid any activities that are done lying on the back, such as sit-ups	• Try not to exercise for longer than 15–20 minutes • Avoid upper-body exercises for CABG patients until fully healed

General precautions
• If angina occurs before or during activity or at rest, stop and follow standard nitrate protocol;* do not start activity again; call emergency services if needed.
• Make sure the client can recognise their symptoms, and know how to administer medication before doing activity.
• Do not supervise individuals in this category if not suitably qualified (BACR is the minimum required).

* Nitrates are prescribed medication only, come as a tablet or spray and are used to give immediate relief of symptoms.

ANGINA

Prior to commencing any cardiac rehabilitation programme, individuals who have been clinically diagnosed with angina should already have undergone an appropriate supervised diagnostic exercise test before being accepted on to an exercise referral programme. The purpose of doing this would have been to establish an appropriate individual range of rate of perceived exertion (RPE) levels using standard angina scale ratings. The other purpose of the test is to establish the upper limits of the individual's heart rate for activity purposes so that those supervising have this information prior to the start of any physical activity programme. Guidelines (as can be seen in table 12.6) have been taken and adapted from a variety of credible sources such as the ACSM and NICE.

MYOCARDIAL INFARCTION (MI)

Table 12.7 shows commonly recommended guidelines for physical activity programming for individuals who have suffered a myocardial infarction within the previous four to six months. This type of activity programming is more commonly known as 'post-MI' exercise. Individuals in this category should already have undergone an appropriate supervised diagnostic

Table 12.7	Physical activity guidelines for individuals who have had an MI	
	Aerobic training	**Strength training**
Mode	• Walking and cycling are good for this condition	• Use a combination of free weights and body weight • Use functional exercises such as standing to sitting squats or lifting tins on and off a shelf • Include mobility of the thoracic spine
Intensity	• Prolonged warm-up and cool-down • Activities between 65 and 90%HRmax • 11–16 RPE	• Use loads up to 40–50% of maximum voluntary contraction • Overload by increasing repetitions then intensity
Duration	• 20–40 minutes of continuous or interval activity • 10 minute warm-up and cool-downs	• Perform 1–3 sets of 10–15 RM • 1–2 minutes' rest between exercises • Balance major muscle groups and upper/lower body
Frequency	• 3 days per week	• 2–3 sessions per week
Precautions	• Set intensity based on results of the walk test (done in clinical environment) • Water-based activities can be hazardous • Avoid any activities that are done lying on the back, such as sit-ups	• Try not to exercise for longer than 15–20 minutes • Avoid upper-body exercises for CABG patients until fully healed • Main muscle groups should be exercised separately

General precautions
• If there is any pain in the chest, neck, throat, arm or back, or any illness such as nausea or vomiting, then call emergency services immediately as suspected MI.
• If this is the case, put individual in a seated position with the head and shoulders supported and the knees bent.
• Do not supervise individuals in this category if not suitably qualified (BACR is the minimum required).

exercise test before being accepted on to an exercise referral programme. This would have been done in order to establish activity levels that would be deemed suitable as a baseline level specifically for the individual, as in the case of those with angina. The guidelines in table 12.7 have been taken and adapted from a variety of credible sources, such as the ACSM and NICE.

PERIPHERAL VASCULAR DISEASE (PVD)

Before any physical activity can be performed with individuals who have PVD, some form of medical clearance should have taken place. The decision for the individual to undertake a level of intensity would have been based on tests such as blood screening, a graded exercise test (GXT) and a thorough physical examination. Guidelines for physical activity relating to sufferers of PVD have been taken and adapted from a variety of credible sources. Table 12.8 shows the recommended guidelines for physical activity programming for those who have had this condition within the previous four to six months.

During physical activity sessions, the supervisor could make use of a pain scale, which is used to rate pain or tiredness felt in the legs when doing any type of activity. This type of scale is known as the 'claudication pain scale', as can be seen in the example in table 12.9. In other words, the scale is used to rate how painful an individual with PVD thinks it is to do a particular activity, and in all

Table 12.8	Physical activity guidelines for individuals who have PVD	
	Aerobic training	**Strength training**
Mode	• Intermittent walking or cycling	• Use a combination of free weights and body weight • Use functional exercises such as standing to sitting squats or lifting tins on and off a shelf • Include mobility of the thoracic spine
Intensity	• Prolonged warm-up and cool-down • 40–70% of the graded exercise test value	• Use loads up to 40–50% of maximum voluntary contraction • Overload by increasing repetitions then intensity
Duration	• 20–40 minutes per session • Done as short periods of activity with rest between	• Perform 3 sets of 10–15 RM • 1–2 minutes' rest between exercises • Balance major muscle groups and upper/lower body
Frequency	• 3–5 days per week	• 2–3 sessions per week • Encourage other forms of exercise
Precaution	• Exercising in the cold can exacerbate the condition	• Try not to exercise for longer than 15–20 minutes

General precautions
• Avoid too much pain during activities.
• No more than level 2 on the claudication pain scale.

Table 12.9	Claudication pain scale
Level	Perception
0	No claudication pain
1	Initial, minimal pain
2	Moderate, bothersome pain
3	Intense pain
4	Maximal pain, cannot continue

cases the individual should be asked to stop before they reach level of 3 on the scale.

There are several training providers that deliver British Association of Cardiac Rehabilitation (BACR) phase IV qualifications, as mentioned earlier. Generally speaking, the courses are practically based and cover both theory and practical implementation of submaximal exercise tests and their application to exercise prescription for individuals with heart disease. The courses tend to be aimed mainly at health and exercise professionals who are either directly involved in or support in the assessment of exercise capacity, and/or advise and prescribe exercise and activity in clinical population groups such as cardiac/pulmonary rehabilitation and claudication programmes (e.g. physiotherapists, exercise instructors, sports scientists, exercise physiologists). Courses normally include instruction for participants on how to carry out typical testing procedures, and then how to apply the test results to exercise and physical activity guidance and prescription. Typical tests that are normally covered on the courses include:

- the 6-minute walk test;
- the incremental shuttle walk test;
- cycle ergometry testing and
- the Chester step test.

RECOMMENDED READING

Ades, P.A., Waldmann, M.L., Poehlman, E.T., Gray, P., Horton, E.D., Horton, E.S. & LeWinter, M.M. (1993) Exercise conditioning in older coronary patients. Submaximal lactate response and endurance capacity. *Circulation*, 88(2): 572–577

American College of Sports Medicine (2009a) *ACSM's exercise management for persons with chronic diseases and disabilities* (3rd edn). Champaign, IL: Human Kinetics

American College of Sports Medicine (2009b) *ACSM's guidelines for exercise testing and prescription* (8th edn). London: Lippincott Williams & Wilkins

Beaglehole, R., Irwin, A. & Prentice, T. (2004) *The World Health Report 2004 – changing history*. Geneva, Switzerland: WHO Press

Boie, E.T. (2005) Initial evaluation of chest pain. *Emergency Medicine Clinics of North America*, 23(4): 937–957

Braunwald, E. (1992) *Heart disease* (4th edn). Philadelphia, PA: W.B. Saunders

British Heart Foundation (2004) *Coronary heart disease statistics*. University of Oxford: Department of Public Health

Canto, J.G., Goldberg, R.J., Hand, M.M., Bonow, R.O., Sopko, G., Pepine, C.J. & Long, T. (2007) Symptom presentation of women with acute coronary syndromes: Myth versus reality. *Archives of International Medicine*, 167(22): 2405–2413

Department of Health (2000) *Coronary heart disease: National service framework for coronary heart disease – modern standards and service models*. London: DH

Erhardt, L., Herlitz, J., Bossaert, L., Halinen, M., Keltai, M., Koster, R., Marcassa, C., Quinn, T. & van Weert, H. (2002) Task force on the management of chest pain. *European Heart Journal*, 23(15): 1153–1176

Fowkes, F.G., Housley, E., Cawood, E.H., Macintyre, C.C., Ruckley, C.V. & Prescott, R.J. (1991) Edinburgh Artery Study: Prevalence of asymptomatic and symptomatic peripheral arterial disease in the general population. *International Journal of Epidemiology*, 20(2): 384–392

Guyton, A.C. (2006) *Textbook of medical physiology* (11th edn). Philadelphia, PA: Elsevier Saunders

Hiatt, W., Hoag, S. & Hamman, R. (1995) Effect of diagnostic criteria on the prevalence of peripheral arterial disease. *Circulation*, 91: 1472–1479

Hombach, V., Höher, M., Kochs, M., Eggeling, T., Schmidt, A., Höpp, H.W. & Hilger, H.H. (1998) Pathophysiology of unstable angina pectoris: Correlations with coronary angioscopic imaging. *European Heart Journal*, 9(N): 40–45

Jolliffe, J.A., Rees, K., Taylor, R.S., Thompson, D., Oldridge, N. & Ibrahim, S. (2001) Exercise-based rehabilitation for coronary heart disease. *Cochrane Database of Systematic Reviews*, (1): CD001800

Kannel, W.B. (1986) Silent myocardial ischemia and infarction: Insights from the Framingham Study. *Cardiology Clinics*, 4(4): 583–591

Manson, J.E., Greenland, P., LaCroix, A.Z., Stefanick, M.L., Mouton, C.P., Oberman, A., Perri, M.G., Sheps, D.S., Pettinger, M.B. & Siscovick, D.S. (2002) Walking compared with vigorous exercise for the prevention of cardiovascular events in women. *New England Journal of Medicine*, 347: 716–725

Manson, J.E., Hu, F.B., Rich-Edwards, J.W., Colditz, G.A., Stampfer, M.J., Willett, W.C., Speizer, F.E. & Hennekens, C.H. (1999) A prospective study of walking as compared with vigorous exercise in the prevention of coronary heart disease in women. *New England Journal of Medicine*, 341: 650–658

McDermott, M.M. (2009) Treadmill exercise and resistance training in patients with peripheral arterial disease with and without intermittent claudication. *Journal of the American Medical Association*, 301(2): 165–174

Morris, C.K. & Froelicher, V.F. (1993) Cardiovascular benefits of physical activity. *Sports Medicine*, 16: 222–236

National Heart Lung and Blood Institute (n.d.) Angina. Available online at: www.nhlbi.nih.gov/health/dci/Diseases/Angina/Angina_SignsAndSymptoms.html (accessed 28 April 2010)

NHS Information Centre, Lifestyle Statistics (2009) *Statistics on obesity, physical activity and diet: England, February 2009*. London: NHS Information Centre for Health and Social Care

Peel, C. & Mossberg, K.A. (1995) Effects of cardiovascular medications on exercise responses. *Physical Therapy*, 75(5): 387–396

Scottish Intercollegiate Guidelines Network (2002) *Cardiac rehabilitation: A national clinical guideline*. SIGN publication volume 57. Edinburgh: SIGN

Selig, S.E. & Hare, D.L. (2006) Evidence-based approach to exercise prescription in chronic heart failure. *British Journal of Sports Medicine*, 41: 407–408

Tanasescu, M., Leitzmann, M.F., Rimm, E.B., Willett, W.C., Stampfer, M.J. & Hu, F.B. (2002) Exercise type and intensity in relation to coronary heart disease in men. *Journal of the American Medical Association*, 288: 1994–2000

Thygesen, K., Alpert, J.S. & White, H.D. (2007) Universal definition of myocardial infarction. *European Heart Journal*, 28(20): 2525–2538

Walther, C., Gielen, S. & Hambrecht, R. (2004) The effect of exercise training on endothelial function in cardiovascular disease in humans. *Exercise Sports Science Reviews*, 32: 129–134

Wells, B.G., Dipiro, J.T., Schwinghammer, T.L. & Dipiro, C.V. (2009) *Pharmacotherapy handbook* (7th edn). New York: McGraw-Hill

Wenger, N.K. & Hellerstein, H.K. (1992) *Rehabilitation of the coronary patient* (3rd edn). New York: Churchill Livingstone

White, H.D. & Chew, D.P. (2008) Acute myocardial infarction. *Lancet*, 372 (9638): 570–584

USEFUL WEBSITES

British Heart Foundation – www.bhf.org.uk

Cochrane Collaboration (Cochrane Reviews) – www.cochrane.org

Department of Health – www.dh.gov.uk

National Heart Lung and Blood Institute – www.nhlbi.nih.gov

NHS Information Centre for Health and Social Care – www.ic.nhs.uk

Scottish Intercollegiate Guidelines Network – www.sign.ac.uk

World Health Organization – www.who.int/en

STROKE

13

KEYPOINTS

- A stroke is something that affects brain function quickly and lasts more than a day.
- Strokes occur when blood flow to the brain is obstructed.
- It is commonly agreed that there are two main types of stroke: ischemic and haemorrhagic.
- It is already the second leading cause of death in the western world after heart disease, and is thought to be responsible for around 10% of deaths worldwide (an estimated 16 million first-time stroke patients and 5.7 million stroke deaths).
- It is estimated that about 150,000 individuals have a stroke in the UK each year, and there are over 67,000 deaths as a result of this.
- Stroke is also considered to be a major risk as it is the third most common cause of death in England and Wales, after heart disease and cancer.
- Stroke accounts for 9% of all deaths in men and 13% of deaths in women in the UK.
- For every individual who has a stroke in the UK, the cost to the NHS is £15,000 over five years; when informal care costs are included, this increases to around £29,000.
- Physical activity has been associated with a reduced risk of stroke.
- Moderately active individuals are less likely to have a stroke or die of stroke-related causes than individuals with low activity levels.

WHAT IS IT?

The World Health Organization (WHO) has defined a stroke as 'rapidly developing clinical signs of local or global disturbance of cerebral function with symptoms lasting more than 24 hours or leading to death, with no apparent cause other than vascular origin' – in other words, something that affects brain functions quickly and lasts for more than a day. A 'stroke' is also known as a 'cerebral vascular accident' (CVA), although this term is becoming less common. Stroke is a major cause of death and permanent disability as it is a condition that directly affects the brain. Strokes occur when,

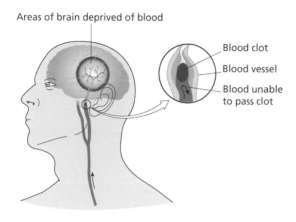

Areas of brain deprived of blood

Blood clot

Blood vessel

Blood unable to pass clot

Figure 13.1 Blockage in an artery to the brain

for some particular reason, blood flow to the brain is obstructed. It is commonly agreed that there are two main types or categories of stroke – those known as 'ischemic' and those known as 'haemorrhagic' strokes (see fig 13.2). In simple terms, ischemic stroke is caused by the blockage of an artery that supplies blood to the brain, as can be seen in fig 13.1. This has the effect of reducing the blood flow and hence the amount of oxygen getting to the brain (which is known as ischemia). Hippocrates (460 to 370 BC) was the first to describe the phenomenon of sudden paralysis that is often associated with a stroke.

In simple terms, haemorrhagic stroke is caused when ruptured blood vessels in the brain cause bleeding (haemorrhage) around the site of the rupture. The amount of bleeding depends on factors such as the degree of the rupture and the blood pressure of the individual. As well as these two types of stroke, there is also an event called a transient ischemic attack (TIA), or mini-stroke. In a TIA, arterial blockage in the brain occurs only briefly but can resolve itself without causing any brain tissue death. Even though only about 10% of ischemic strokes are preceded by a TIA, about 40% of individuals who have a TIA then go on to have a stroke at some stage in their lives.

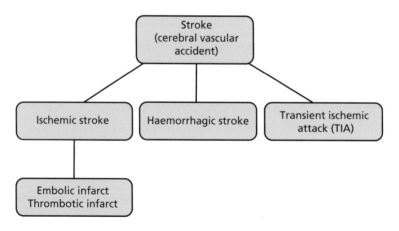

Figure 13.2 Overview of stroke types

ISCHEMIC STROKE

Approximately 80% of all strokes that occur are of the ischemic type. The associated blockage normally develops in one of the major blood vessels on the surface of the brain (this is known as a large-vessel infarct) or can develop in small blood vessels deep within the brain (this is known as a small-vessel infarct). Infarcts that result in ischemic stroke can do so in different ways, therefore there are various classifications of ischemic stroke, which include embolic infarct, thrombotic infarct and lacunar infarct.

- **Embolic infarct:** This occurs when a blood clot (known as an embolism) forms somewhere in the body but breaks free and travels through the bloodstream, where it can become lodged and obstruct the blood flow to the brain. When a clot becomes lodged somewhere in the heart it is known as a 'cardiac embolism'. It is thought that this type of infarct accounts for about 20–30% of all ischemic strokes.
- **Thrombotic infarct:** This type of infarct occurs when a blood clot forms in one of the arteries that supply the brain. When this occurs, after a period of time the clot build-up can lead to death of the surrounding tissues. The clot usually forms due to a build-up of plaque in the arteries (this is known as atherosclerosis). If the clot breaks off and travels through the body then it becomes an embolism.
- **Lacunar infarct:** This is the name given to an infarct when there is blockage of one of the deep penetrating arteries in the brain. It is thought that the main cause of the blockage is due to 'atheroma' or fatty deposits within the artery. It is estimated that this type of infarct accounts for about 25% of all ischemic strokes

HAEMORRHAGIC STROKE

This type of stroke occurs when a blood vessel in the brain ruptures (tears or splits) and bleeds into any surrounding tissue, leading to an accumulation of blood anywhere in the skull cavity. As a result of this, the bleeding has the effect of compressing blood vessels and tissues in the surrounding area, which in turn deprives surrounding tissue of oxygen, leading to a stroke. Unfortunately a haemorrhagic stroke usually affects a large area of the brain and as such carries a high risk of death. If the bleeding occurs within the brain it is known as 'intra-axial haemorrhage', but if the bleeding occurs between the inner surface of the skull and the outside of the brain it is known as 'extra-axial haemorrhage'. There are subtypes of extra-axial bleeding, but these are beyond the scope of this book.

PREVALENCE

Many sources agree that stroke could soon be the most common cause of death worldwide. It is already considered to be the second leading cause of death in the western world, after heart disease, and is thought to be responsible for around 10% of all deaths worldwide (an estimated 16 million first-time stroke patients and 5.7 million stroke deaths). It is generally estimated that about 150,000 individuals in the UK have a stroke each year and that there are over 67,000 deaths as a result of this. As far as the UK is concerned, stroke is considered to be a major risk as it is the third most common cause of death in England and Wales, after heart disease and cancer. According to the British Heart Foundation, stroke accounts for about 9% of all deaths in men and about 13% of all deaths in women in the UK. In a report that was published in 2005 by

the Department of Health, it was stated that approximately 110,000 strokes and a further 20,000 transient ischemic attacks (TIAs) occurred in England every year and, furthermore, that there were at least 300,000 individuals in England alone living with moderate to severe disabilities as a result of stroke. The Department of Health also reported that for every individual who has a stroke in the UK, the cost to the National Health Service (NHS) is around £15,000 over five years; when informal care costs are included, this increases to around £29,000. A report by Allender and colleagues in 2008 expanded further on stroke care costs to the NHS. They estimated that about £3 billion a year was spent in direct care costs by the NHS, and a further £5 billion more was attributed to the wider economy due to mortality and morbidity and informal care costs (costs of home nursing and care borne by patients' families). This results in a total cost to the UK economy of about £8 billion per year.

SYMPTOMS

Stroke symptoms typically start very suddenly (over seconds to minutes) and depend on the area of the brain that is affected. The more extensive the area of brain that is affected, the more functions are likely to be lost. Most forms of stroke are not associated with headaches but they can occur, although infrequently, with specific types. As strokes are considered to be medical emergencies that require immediate medical attention, it is important that symptoms or warning signs are recognised as quickly as possible as they are often difficult to identify. To help recognise the symptoms of a stroke, various systems over the years have been proposed. One of the earliest recommended recognition tools was to get the patient to raise both arms and to watch and see if one of the arms involuntarily drifted down, indicating a problem if it did. More recently, systems such as FAST (face, arm, speech and time) have been widely proposed (see table 13.1). The FAST system is advocated by many international organisations, such as the Department of Health, the Stroke Association and the American Stroke Association. This particular stroke recognition system is designed to be used by anyone so that if the individual suspected of having a stroke has difficulty with *any one* of the FAST tasks, emergency services should be called immediately and symptoms described to the individual on the phone.

Table 13.1		Symptoms of a stroke
F	Face	• Ask the individual to smile • One side of the face can be numb and drop, and the mouth can drool • Vision in one or both eyes can be lost
A	Arms	• Ask the individual to raise *both* arms • Paralysis can occur on one side of the body
S	Speech	• Ask the individual to speak a simple sentence • Slurred speech is usually an indication • Confusion and difficulty responding often occur
T	Time	• If the individual cannot respond to any of the above it is time to call 999

RISK FACTORS

According to the American Heart Association, the risk factors for ischemic stroke can be grouped into those that are non-modifiable and modifiable, as described in table 13.2.

Most of the risk factors relating to strokes can be avoided by prevention measures. Although it is

Table 13.2	Modifiable and non-modifiable risk factors for ischemic stroke
Non-modifiable risk factors	**Description**
Gender	In most age groups, more men than women have a stroke in a given year, but more than half of total stroke deaths occur in women; the use of birth control pills and pregnancy can increase the risk for women
Age	95% of all strokes occur in individuals around the age of 45 years and older, and two-thirds of strokes occur in those over the age of 65; the chance of having a stroke approximately doubles for each decade of life after the age of 55
Family or individual history of stroke	Risk is considered to be greater if a parent, grandparent, sister or brother has previously had a stroke or if the individual has had a previous stroke.
Modifiable risk factors	**Description**
High blood pressure	High blood pressure (hypertension) accounts for about 35–50% of total stroke risk, and it has been shown that even a small blood pressure reduction (5–6 mmHg systolic or 2–3 mmHg diastolic) would result in around 40% fewer strokes (both ischemic and haemorrhagic)
Atrial fibrillation	Those individuals with atrial fibrillation (irregular heart beat) have a slightly increased risk of stroke (see http://en.wikipedia.org/wiki/Stroke–cite_note-AFIB-53); with this particular condition the heart does not beat effectively, which can lead to blood pooling and clotting; if a clot subsequently breaks off then enters the bloodstream and lodges in an artery leading to the brain, this can result in an embolic stroke
Smoking	In recent years, many studies have shown cigarette smoking to be a risk factor for stroke; for instance, nicotine and carbon monoxide in cigarette smoke can damage artery walls, allowing clots to form; it is these clots that can then result in various types of infarct
High cholesterol	Although the research is not fully clear, generally speaking individuals with high blood cholesterol have an increased risk of stroke; also, it appears that low HDL (good) cholesterol is a risk factor for stroke in men
Diabetes	Diabetes is considered to be an independent risk factor for stroke (2–3 times more likely); many individuals with diabetes also have high blood pressure, high blood cholesterol and are overweight or obese, which increases their risk even more
Narrowing of arteries (arterial stenosis)	Arteries can become narrowed (known as stenosis) as a result, among other things, of fatty deposits from atherosclerosis (plaque build-up on the artery walls); if this occurs it can increase the risk of stroke

quite a complex issue, the following general recommendations can be followed to help reduce the overall risk:

- do not smoke
- exercise regularly
- limit intake of salt, alcohol and saturated fat
- use safety devices such as airbags, seatbelts, child safety seats and protective headgear.

DIAGNOSIS

Although symptoms can be recognised and acted upon, diagnosis is always done by a qualified individual, which includes a physical (and neurological) examination to evaluate the level of consciousness, sensation and function (visual, motor, language). This is important as it can help to determine the cause, location and extent of the stroke as quickly as possible to prevent further damage to the brain. Blood tests and imaging procedures (e.g. CT scan, ultrasound, MRI) are often carried out in order to do this.

PHYSICAL ACTIVITY BENEFITS

With regard to the prevention of stroke, being inactive, obese or both can increase an individual's risk of high blood pressure, high blood cholesterol, diabetes, heart disease and stroke. It is important therefore that regular physical activity be adopted as early and as regularly as possible to lower the risk of stroke (and other conditions). The long-term goals of treatment for individuals who have had a stroke often include rehabilitation, which includes physical activity. This can help to prevent the further occurrence of strokes. Table 13.3 gives an overview of the initial treatment, rehabilitation and prognosis for both types of stroke.

In terms of published studies, physical activity has been associated with a reduced risk of stroke. For instance, a review of 18 studies that was carried out found that moderately active individuals were 17% less likely to have a stroke or die of stroke-related causes than were individuals with low activity (25% for highly active individuals). In relation to both types of strokes, studies such as

Table 13.3	Initial treatment, rehabilitation and prognosis for both types of stroke		
	Initial treatment	**Rehabilitation**	**Prognosis**
Ischemic stroke	This involves removing the blockage and restoring blood flow	Often includes physical therapy, speech therapy and occupational therapy	Approximately 70% regain independence and 10% recover almost completely; approximately 25% die as a result of the stroke
Haemorrhagic stroke	This usually requires surgery to relieve the pressure within the skull caused by bleeding	Often includes physical therapy, speech therapy and occupational therapy	The location of a haemorrhagic stroke is the important factor, but this type is generally worse than ischemic stroke

the nurses' health study by Hu *et al.* (2000), showed that women in the highest activity category experienced only half the risk of ischemic stroke as the least active category. Other studies, including the physicians' health study for men by Lee *et al.* (1999), indicate that physical activity may also be beneficial in preventing haemorrhagic stroke. In terms of using physical activity for rehabilitation of those that suffered a stroke, a study by Mead and colleagues in 2007 used 66 post-stroke patients to undergo three physical activity sessions for 12 weeks and found great benefits as a result. For guidelines, see table 13.4.

Table 13.4	Physical activity guidelines for individuals who have suffered a stroke	
	Aerobic training	**Strength training**
Mode	• Large-muscle activities (e.g. walking, treadmill, stationary cycle, combined arm-leg ergometry, arm ergometry, seated stepper)	• Use a combination of free weights and body weight • Use functional exercises such as standing to sitting squats or lifting tins on and off a shelf (called activities of daily living, or ADLs)
Intensity	• Prolonged warm-up and cool-down • Exercise at a rate of 50–80%HRmax • 8–14 RPE	• Use loads up to 40–50% of maximum voluntary contraction • Overload by increasing repetitions then intensity
Duration	• 20–60 minutes of continuous or interval exercise, or • Multiple 10-minute sessions	• Perform 1–3 sets of 10–15 RM • 1–2 minutes' rest between exercises • Balance major muscle groups and upper/lower body
Frequency	• 3–7 days per week	• 2–3 days per week • Encourage other forms of exercise
Precautions	• Set intensity based on results of the walk test	• Try not to exercise for longer than 15–20 minutes

General precautions
- If any problems occur, such as walking problems, facial or body weakness and affected speech, then stop immediately and use the FAST procedure as described in table 13.1.
- Try to pick times when facilities are not crowded and noisy.
- Group sessions might help social interaction.
- Provide written instructions to aid understanding.

PHYSICAL ACTIVITY GUIDELINES

Following a stroke, individuals tend to become extremely deconditioned and in some cases have some degree of impairment such as hemiplegia and spasticity. This loss of function can also affect the individual psychologically, therefore it is very important that a programme of physical activity is started as soon as possible. The goals of individuals who have suffered impairment may be as simple as improving range of motion and performance of daily living tasks and an improvement in well-being.

RECOMMENDED READING

Allender, S., Scarborough, P., Peto, V., Rayner, M., Leal, J., Luengo-Fernandez, R. & Gray, A. (2008) *European cardiovascular disease statistics*. Brussels: European Heart Network

American College of Sports Medicine (2009a) *ACSM's exercise management for persons with chronic diseases and disabilities* (3rd edn). Champaign, IL: Human Kinetics

American College of Sports Medicine (2009b) *ACSM's guidelines for exercise testing and prescription* (8th edn). London: Lippincott Williams & Wilkins

American Heart Association (2010) Stroke risk factors. Available online at: www.heart.org (accessed 22 July 2010)

British Heart Foundation Health Promotion Research Group (2005) *Coronary heart disease statistics*. University of Oxford: Department of Public Health

Chalela, J.A., Kidwell, C.S., Nentwich, L.M., Luby, M., Butman, J.A., Demchuk, A.M., Hill, M.D., Patronas, N., Latour, L. & Warach, S. (2007) Magnetic resonance imaging and computed tomography in emergency assessment of patients with suspected acute stroke: A prospective comparison. *Lancet*, 369(9558): 293–298

Deb, P., Sharma, S. & Hassan, K.M. (2010) Pathophysiologic mechanisms of acute ischemic stroke:

An overview with emphasis on therapeutic significance beyond thrombolysis. *Pathophysiology*, 17(3): 197–218

Department of Health (2005) *Reducing brain damage: Faster access to better stroke care*. London: The Stationery Office

Donnan, G.A., Fisher, M., Macleod, M. & Davis, S.M. (2008) Stroke. *Lancet*, 371(9624): 1612–1623

Ederle, J. & Brown, M.M. (2006) The evidence for medicine versus surgery for carotid stenosis. *European Journal of Radiology*, 60(1): 3–7

Ederle, J., Featherstone, R.L. & Brown, M.M. (2007) Percutaneous transluminal angioplasty and stenting for carotid artery stenosis. *Cochrane Database of Systematic Reviews*, 4: CD 000515

Feigin, V.L. (2005) Stroke epidemiology in the developing world. *Lancet*, 365(9478): 2160–2161

Goldstein, L.B. & Simel, D.L. (2005) Is this patient having a stroke? *Journal of the American Medical Association*, 293(19): 2391–2402

Hankey, G.J. (1999) Smoking and risk of stroke. *Journal of Cardiovascular Risk*, 6(4): 207–211

Harbison, J., Massey, A., Barnett, L., Hodge, D. & Ford, G.A. (1999) Rapid ambulance protocol for acute stroke. *Lancet*, 353(9168): 1935

Hu, F.B., Stampfer, M.J., Colditz, G.A., Ascherio, A., Rexrode, K.M., Willett, W.C. & Manson, J.E. (2000) Physical activity and risk of stroke in women. *Journal of the American Medical Association*, 283: 2961–2967

Intercollegiate Working Party for Stroke (2000) *National clinical guidelines for stroke*. London: Royal College of Physicians

Kidwell, C.S. & Warach, S. (2003) Acute ischemic cerebrovascular syndrome: Diagnostic criteria. *Stroke*, 34(12): 2995–2998

Lee, C.D., Folsom, A.R. & Blair, S.N. (2003) Physical activity and stroke risk: A meta-analysis. *Stroke*, 34: 2475–2481

Lee, I.M., Hennekens, C.H., Berger, K., Buring, J.E. & Manson, J.E. (1999) Exercise and risk of stroke in male physicians. *Stroke*, 30: 1–6

Mead, G.E., Greig, C.A., Cunningham, I., Lewis, S.J., Dinan, S.M., Saunders, D.M., Fitzsimons, C. & Young, A. (2007) Stroke: A randomised trial of exercise or relaxation. *Journal of American Geriatrics Society*, 55: 892–899

Mohr, J.P., Choi, D., Grotta, J. & Wolf, P. (2004) *Stroke: Pathophysiology, diagnosis, and management* (4th edn). New York: Churchill Livingstone

National Collaborating Centre for Chronic Conditions (2008) *Stroke: National clinical guideline for diagnosis and initial management of acute stroke and transient ischaemic attack (TIA).* London: Royal College of Physicians

Prospective Studies Collaboration (1995) Cholesterol, diastolic blood pressure, and stroke: 13,000 strokes in 450,000 individuals in 45 prospective cohorts. *Lancet*, 346(8991–8992): 1647–1653

Reynolds, K., Lewis, B., Nolen, J.D., Kinney, G.L., Sathya, B. & He, J. (2003) Alcohol consumption and risk of stroke: A meta-analysis. *Journal of the American Medical Association*, 289(5): 579–588

Rudd, A.G., Irwin, P., Rutledge, Z., Lowe, D., Morris, R. & Pearson, M.G. (1999) The national sentinel audit of stroke: A tool for raising standards of care. *Journal of the Royal College of Physicians London*, 33: 460–464

Scottish Intercollegiate Guidelines Network (SIGN 78) (2004) *Management of patients with stroke: Identification and management of dysphagia. A national clinical guideline.* Edinburgh: Scottish Intercollegiate Guidelines Network Royal College of Physicians

Scottish Stroke Care Audit (2006) Winter 2001 Stroke incidence and risk factors in a population based cohort study. *Office of National Statistics Health Statistics Quarterly* (12)

Sims, N.R. & Muyderman, H. (2009) Mitochondria, oxidative metabolism and cell death in stroke. *Biochimica et Biophysica Acta*, 1802(1): 80–91

Stam, J. (2005) Thrombosis of the cerebral veins and sinuses. *New England Journal of Medicine*, 352(17): 1791–1798

Thomson, R. (2009) Evidence based implementation of complex interventions. *British Medical Journal*, 339: B3124

Wolf, P.A., Abbott, R.D. & Kannel, W.B. (1987) Atrial fibrillation: A major contributor to stroke in the elderly. The Framingham Study. *Archives of Internal Medicine*, 147(9): 1561–1564

USEFUL WEBSITES

American Heart Association – www.heart.org
British Heart Foundation – www.bhf.org.uk
Cochrane Collaboration (Cochrane Reviews) – www.cochrane.org
Department of Health – www.dh.gov.uk
National Institute of Neurological Disorders and Stroke – www.ninds.nih.gov
Royal College of Physicians – www.rcplondon.ac.uk
Scottish Intercollegiate Guidelines Network – www.sign.ac.uk
Stroke Association – www.stroke.org.uk
UK National Statistics (health statistics) – www.statistics.gov.uk

// YOUNGER AGE 14

WHAT IS IT?

It can be quite confusing when talking about the different stages of childhood as there are many terms that are often used to describe children before they become adults. To help clarify this and provide standardisation in terms of delivery supervision, table 14.1 gives a description of terms that are used throughout the different stages of childhood up to adulthood.

The development of a human being can be broadly categorised into two distinctly different areas, that of 'physiological' (this means anything to do with the body) and that of 'psychological'

Table 14.1	Terms related to stages of development
Stage of development	**Description**
Infancy	This term normally refers only to the first year of a child's life
Childhood	The term childhood should be used from the age of 1 year up to the age of puberty (typically between 10 and 14 years)
Puberty	This is when the development of secondary sex characteristics and the capability of sexual reproduction occur, usually between the ages mentioned above
Adolescence	This is the term used to describe the range from puberty to the completion of growth and development (adulthood)

(anything to do with the mind). Even though there are many more areas of physiological and psychological development that can be explored, for the purpose of this book, only the areas of skeletal (bone), muscular, cardiovascular development, self-esteem and exercise behaviour will be briefly covered.

SKELETAL DEVELOPMENT

It is well known that bones do not grow at a steady rate throughout life. The fastest rate of growth of bone is typically within the first two years of life when a child can reach up to half of their full-grown adult height. Generally speaking, bone growth can continue until the early 20s at an average rate of about 2 inches per year, but is usually different for boys and girls. Girls generally mature physiologically about 2–2.5 years earlier than boys. Growth spurts (a period when growth appears to be quicker) tend to occur at different times throughout life for boys and girls. In the case of girls, for instance, the main period of growth spurt typically occurs between the ages of 10 and 13. For boys, however, the main period of growth spurt typically occurs around the ages of 12–14. As bones are still growing at this age, this often means that children are more susceptible to certain injuries as they do not have the bone strength needed to cope with the sustained high-impact activities that children often take part in. In relation to bone growth during childhood, there are many nutrients that are required in the diet, such as calcium, vitamin C and phosphorous. As well as dietary factors affecting bone growth, hormones can also affect it at different times throughout life. Growth hormone and testosterone are just two of the hormones that can affect the rate of growth, particularly around puberty.

MUSCULAR DEVELOPMENT

As with skeletal growth, the muscles in the body also grow at irregular rates. It is generally thought that the number of muscle fibres is genetically determined and that growth of a muscle is due to enlargement of the fibres in the muscles, and not due to splitting or increasing the number of muscle fibres. The enlargement of muscle fibres (known as 'hypertrophy') makes them thicker, but muscle fibres can also get longer. Generally speaking, at puberty, boys tend to have a faster rate of muscle growth than girls due to increased levels of the hormone testosterone, which helps to stimulate muscle growth. With certain types of training (and the right genetics) boys' muscle mass can peak at about 50% of body weight around the age

165

of 18 to 25 years, whereas girls' muscle mass peaks at about 40% of body weight around the age of 16 to 20 years.

CARDIOVASCULAR DEVELOPMENT

Children cannot pump the same amount of blood around the body in the same time period as adults can because they have smaller heart chambers and lower blood volume than that of adults. This means that stroke volume (the amount of blood pumped out of the heart each beat) and cardiac output (the total amount pumped in 1 minute) are lower in children. For this reason, a child typically needs to work harder than an adult as they can supply only a fraction of the oxygen requirements of muscles in comparison to adults. In other words, children are less efficient than adults. In relation to the pulmonary system, development of the air sacs in the lungs (alveoli) is virtually complete by the age of 6. From this age onwards the alveoli increase in size. Relative to adults, the work of breathing during physical exertion is higher in children. As a measure of aerobic fitness, VO_2 increases from about the age of 6 through to adolescence in males and females, where females then tend to plateau and males continue to increase. The energy requirement for walking and running is higher in young children than in adults, which is possibly due to a greater running economy in adults. It often appears that older children do not seem to be working as hard as younger children during activities in which they are all participating (assuming fitness levels are reasonably equal). This is because movement becomes more efficient with age. This is important, as younger children can normally sustain high levels of exercise or activity for only short periods of time even though this will develop as they get older and fitter.

SELF-ESTEEM

As children develop they form an opinion or an image of themselves normally based on how others see them (not just in sporting situations but in everyday life as well). This opinion of ourselves is what is generally known as 'self-esteem'. Even though the concept is not fully understood, it has been shown that there are many factors that can influence an individual's perception of self-esteem. Figure 14.1 shows an example of just some of the possibilities that have a direct influence on self-esteem. It is generally thought that exposing the child to some sort of success, in relation to sports or activities, on a regular basis, plays a major role in helping to build the confidence of young children, which can then result in a positive influence on their self-esteem. In terms of supervising physical activity, it is critical therefore to provide young children with a positive and encouraging environment in which they can develop and continue to participate.

EXERCISE BEHAVIOUR

The way that children participate (or not as the case may be) in physical activity or exercise is sometimes referred to as 'exercise behaviour'. There are many possible reasons why children would start participating in a particular activity and then choose to either continue (adhere) with that activity or just drop out. Children might have more than one reason to take up and maintain a particular activity, and it is a common belief that these reasons change over a period of time. Much research has been done in this particular area; table 14.2 lists just some of the more common reasons why children might want to join in an activity and keep coming back to take part.

There are many proposed theories relating to

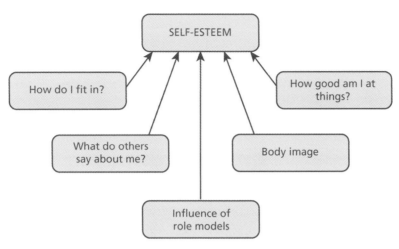

Figure 14.1 Factors that can affect self-esteem

Table 14.2	Common reasons for children participating in and adhering to activities	
Take up	**Come back**	
Looks fun	Enjoyment	
Join in with friends	Varied activities	
Join in with family	Self-esteem	
Play at school	Social	
Don't want to be left out	Help others	
Make new fiends	Role model	
My role model does this	I am good at this	

changing exercise or physical activity behaviour. These theories are better known as 'behavioural change models'. However, these models tend to relate more to older children and adults, therefore those supervising physical activity for children should just be aware of the main reasons why children would keep coming back and try to facilitate this. One of the main reasons children adhere to exercise or specific activities appears to be the enjoyment factor, or simply having fun. For many years psychologists have known about

and studied the link between having fun and arousal. This potential link makes a difference in sport and physical activity as it has been shown that when arousal levels in children are low, they generally get bored very easily and stop participating in the activity, whereas when arousal levels are high, children tend to enjoy themselves and keep participating. It should be pointed out however that if arousal levels become too high, then in certain situations this can cause fear and anxiety.

PREVALENCE: HEALTH SURVEY

Much research has been done over the years relating to leisure-time activity and sedentary entertainment. For example, in a study in the UK undertaken by the Health Education Authority (HEA) in 1998 (*Young and active? Young people and health-enhancing physical activity: Evidence and implications*), it was reported that approximately 75% of the 11–16-year-old children that were questioned watched television for at least 2 hours per day, and the remainder watched in excess of 4 hours per day. The report also suggested that computers, computer games and other alternative media activities took up a large proportion of sedentary behaviour with around 10% of the 11–16 year olds playing computer games for in excess of 10 hours per week. As the HEA report was extensive and it is beyond the scope of this book to describe it in full, some other interesting figures and statements from the report are listed below.

- Children expend approximately 600 kcals (it can take up to an hour to burn this much) per day fewer than did children 50 years ago.
- Since the mid-1980s the average number of miles walked per year has fallen by over 20%.
- Since the mid-1980s the average number of miles cycled has decreased by more than 10%.
- Since the mid-1980s the number of children travelling to school by car has doubled.

In relation to research in the same area, in 2005 the Department of Health (DH) published a report which suggested that children in the UK now tend to walk or cycle less and less, and increasingly rely on cars as a means of transportation. The DH also stated that children are now tending to opt out of active leisure pursuits and recreational sports, and are choosing a range of sedentary entertainment such as watching television, playing video games and using computers instead. It is important to note that the DH has stated that physical activity has a significant role to play in contributing to the health and well-being of communities across the whole of the country (the UK). It has also stated that regular exercise and physical activity provide substantial health benefits and reduce the risk of developing overweight and obesity, and all the potential accompanying health defects caused (or made worse) by the conditions. With this in mind, getting children involved in physical activity and exercise can therefore be considered to be of paramount importance as, according to the *Foresight Report* in 2007, by 2050 up to 55% of boys and about 70% of girls could be overweight or obese. The *Health Survey for England 2008* was a report published in 2009 that further expanded on the DH report of 2005. In this report, school children (the age range of all children was 2–15 years) across the country were asked many questions relating to their individual physical activity and sedentary time habits. Some of the younger children needed assistance with the questions, whereas the older children completed the questions themselves. This type of questionnaire is known as a 'self-reported measure'. Even though many questions were asked, a summary of the responses to some of the questions can be seen in table 14.3.

It can be seen from the *Health Survey for England* report that, in general, boys become more active throughout their childhood, whereas girls

Table 14.3	Summary of responses from the 2008 *Health Survey of England*
General question	**Response**
How much physical activity do you do out of school hours?	Based on their responses, a higher proportion of boys than girls aged 2–15 years were classified as meeting the government's recommendations for physical activity, doing at least an hour of at least moderate activity every day (32% for boys and 24% for girls); interestingly, among girls the percentage generally decreased with age, ranging from 35% among girls aged 2 years to 12% among those aged 14 years; however this didn't really happen among boys
How much physical activity did you do last week?	Overall, 95% of boys and girls had participated in some kind of physical activity in the last week; more girls than boys had done some walking (65% for girls and 61% for boys); boys were more likely than girls to have participated in informal activities (90% for boys and 86% for girls) and formal sports (49% for boys and 38% for girls); the average total number of hours of physical activity in the last 7 days was greater for boys than for girls (10.0 for boys and 8.7 for girls); for most children, informal sports and activities were the main part of their activities, but for girls aged 14–15 years, more of their activity came from walking
How much sedentary time do you have out of school hours?	Average total sedentary time was very similar for boys and girls on weekdays (3.4 hours each) and weekend days (4.1 hours and 4.2 hours); average sedentary time generally increased with age; sedentary time was different for weekdays and weekend days – on weekdays, fewer than 10% of those aged 2–9 years were sedentary for six or more hours, rising steeply with age, while at weekends the proportion that were sedentary for 6 or more hours generally increased across all ages, ranging from 8% of boys and girls aged to 2 years to 40% of boys and 41% of girls aged 15 years

tend to become less active, however sedentary time increased throughout childhood for both boys and girls. As self-reported measures are always criticised for not being accurate, the survey also used another measurement tool: a random sample of 1707 children aged 4–15 years were chosen to carry out 'accelerometer' measurements that were compared against their self-reported data. An accelerometer is a device that when worn can accurately track (depending on the type of accelerometer) the amount of movement the person is doing. The accelerometers were worn by the sample of children for at least 10 hours per day on at least four days of the week, and some wore the accelerometer for the full seven days. While results were similar using the different methods of measurement, there was a much larger differentiation between younger and older children using the accelerometer method than with the self-reported method. This suggests that the self-report method may underestimate physical activity in younger children, and overestimate among older children. In a more recent study, published in 2010, Guthold *et al.*

compared levels of physical activity and sedentary behaviour in schoolchildren from 34 countries. The Global School-based Student Health Survey (GSHS), as it was called, was a collection of data by means of a questionnaire from 72,845 schoolchildren between 2003 and 2007. The questionnaire included questions on overall physical activity, walking or biking to school, and on time spent sitting. The results showed that very few of the children engaged in sufficient physical activity. Across all countries, an average of only 23.8% of boys and 15.4% of girls met general recommendations. In more than half of the countries, however, more than one-third of the children spent 3 or more hours per day on sedentary activities (excluding the hours spent sitting at school and doing homework).

PHYSICAL ACTIVITY BENEFITS

As with other populations, there are many potential physiological and psychological benefits related to participation in regular physical activity. Although the exact nature of any physical activity programme can be vastly different and specific to the individual, the benefits to children are similar to those of adults and in general can include the following:

- increased strength and endurance
- enhanced bone formation
- weight management
- reduced anxiety and stress
- improved self-esteem
- minimisation of heart disease risk factors
- skill development
- social interaction.

According to the DH (2004), there is a great deal of evidence for encouraging young people to be physically active, not only for the reason of health benefits but for other factors, such as learning of social skills, developing creative intelligence, stimulating growth and increasing fitness levels. It should be mentioned, however, that because of the ethical problems relating to research undertaken with children, there is relatively little direct evidence (compared with adults) linking physical inactivity in children with childhood health problems, as confirmed by Boreham and Riddoch in 2001. Children are however at risk of certain conditions (such as obesity, diabetes, cardiovascular disease, and impaired bone health and mental health) in later life, for which the risk can be reduced if regular physical activity is maintained throughout childhood. The benefits of regular physical activity related to each of these conditions can be dealt with separately.

OBESITY

The high, and continually rising, levels of overweight and obesity (see chapter 2 for definitions) among children and young people in England have been described in chapter 1. In 2007, approximately 30.3% of boys and 30.7% of girls aged 2–15 years were at least overweight, and 16.8% of boys and 16.1% of girls in this age group were obese. This is a major problem, as according to research such as that by Freedman *et al.* (1999) and Reich *et al.* (2003), children who are obese are more likely to have certain cardiovascular risk factors. Research by McGill and colleagues (2000) also shows that obese children have a higher incidence of premature blocking of arteries (known as atherosclerosis).

As well as the physical problems associated with obesity in children, Gortmaker *et al.* (1993) and Schwimmer *et al.* (2003) showed that obese children are more likely to have social problems and a lower quality of life. The degree to which a lack of regular physical activity is responsible for the rising levels of obesity in children is still unclear, but there are many studies which suggest that less active children are more likely to have excess fat even as early as late infancy. Much has been made of children who spend more time involved in sedentary activities, such as watching television, being more likely to have excess fat. However, this has recently been questioned because of the link between eating more and watching television. There is also an argument that some children, who watch television for what is considered to be too much time, might have different levels of activity for the rest of the day, which will obviously have a different effect on obesity depending on the individual level of activity. What seems to be clear, though, is that regular physical activity is widely recommended for children of all ages as part of an overall scheme to combat and, possibly more importantly, prevent obesity. One of the reasons for this is that it is generally thought that childhood obesity tracks into adulthood, particularly among those children who have one or two obese parents. For example, research such as that by Freedman *et al.* (1999) and Sinaiko *et al.* (1999), has shown that between 26 and 41% of children who are obese at pre-school age and between 42 and 63% of obese school-age children become obese adults, which can increase the risk of poorer health and increased mortality compared with adults who were not obese as children.

DIABETES

It is estimated that, in the UK alone, there are about 1.4 to 1.6 million individuals who have been diagnosed with diabetes (see chapter 3). Reports such as that by the DH in 2004, state that the level of type 2 diabetes in children and adolescents in the UK is steadily increasing. The report also states that, although the numbers at the moment are relatively low, the last 30 years has seen a threefold increase in the number of cases of childhood diabetes. Because of other related health problems such as obesity, increased insulin resistance, disordered lipid profile and elevated blood pressure appearing in children, it is now more likely that overall cases of diabetes will increase. It is widely acknowledged that, in adults, physical inactivity and obesity are considered to be major risk factors for type 2 diabetes. Even though this is not yet fully understood in children, there is a suggestion, by those such as the American Diabetes Society, that the appearance of type 2 diabetes at younger ages may be due to the increase of obesity and the decrease in levels of physical activity.

MENTAL HEALTH

There is a great deal of evidence to show that regular physical activity is important for children's psychological well-being, such as that from Mutrie and Parfitt (1998), who, having investigated the effects of physical activity on mental, social and moral health on behalf of the Health Education Authority (HEA), found positively related benefits. There is a range of current evidence to indicate that regular physical activity programmes can have a generally positive impact on the mental health of young people. Both Fox (2000) and Gruber (1986) took this a stage further to show that sport and exercise can both have positive effects on self-esteem and body image, especially for those children who already have low self-esteem. Unfortunately, the investigations into the effects of physical activity on reducing stress, anxiety and depression have not been as successful, with most showing that there is only a weak effect. With respect to cognitive functioning, in 2003, a researcher by the name of Sibley, working with Etnier, carried out a review of investigations into the effects of physical activity, and found that children with higher physical activity levels were more likely to have better cognitive functioning. This point is often argued, with some saying that this is not the case, but there is evidence, such as the published SPARK project by Sallis *et al.* (1999), which shows that an increase in physical education does not necessarily have detrimental effects on school academic performance (cognitive functioning). In terms of what type of physical activity might provide mental health benefits, research by McCurdy and colleagues in 2010 showed that there are both mental and physical health benefits associated with unstructured, outdoor activities and time spent in natural environments such as parks or other recreational areas. It can be considered, therefore, that these types of activity are crucial for children as a form of physical activity.

CARDIOVASCULAR DISEASE (CVD)

It is generally agreed that CVD is not a disease of childhood, however children who have lower levels of physical activity are more likely to have risk factors for CVD, such as high blood pressure and cholesterol levels. In other words, children with these risk factors are more likely to have CVD later in life. It is important, therefore, that studies such as those by Boreham and Riddoch (2001) and Twisk (2001) have shown that physical activity has a beneficial effect on blood lipid profiles in children. Unfortunately, though, the effects of physical activity on blood pressure have not been found to be as good but some studies do show a beneficial, if weak, association (meaning physical activity can slightly reduce blood pressure). One thing that is clear however is that low levels of aerobic fitness in children are more likely to lead to multiple risk factors for CVD. This can be evidenced as in studies such as those by Riddoch (1998), Twisk (2001) and Wedderkopp *et al.* (2003), which have shown that children with higher levels of physical activity generally have higher levels of aerobic fitness, and those with low levels of aerobic fitness are more likely to have multiple risk factors for CVD. As mentioned earlier, overweight and obesity are thought to be among the main risk factors for the development of CVD. It makes sense, therefore, that if regular physical activity can help to prevent excess weight gain during childhood, then this might also help to reduce the risk of CVD developing later in life.

BONE HEALTH

It is common knowledge that children's bones grow (and increase in bone mineral density) quite quickly in childhood and adolescence, especially around the years of the growth spurt (this is a term used for rapid growth around the ages of 10 to 13 in girls and 12 to 14 in boys). If this growth occurs normally, as it should do, it can reduce the chances of loss of bone mass and the likelihood of osteoporosis (see chapter 9) in later life. As discussed in the chapter on osteoporosis, regular physical activity into the mid-20s is essential to help develop bone mass, with particular importance around the age of puberty. It was also discussed that weight-bearing activities such as jumping, dancing, aerobics, gymnastics, volleyball, racquet sports and soccer are particularly good for increasing bone mineral density. In general, the amount of physical activity that is needed for any kind of benefit appears to be achieved after only a few repetitions of an activity done on a regular basis. It has also been demonstrated that children who do these sorts of physical activities have, on average, 5–15% more bone mineral density than those children who are classed as inactive. According to a wide range of research, such as that by Boreham and Riddoch in 2001, having a higher bone mineral density is considered to be sufficient enough to significantly reduce the risk of osteoporotic fracture if the activities are maintained into older age (as long as the activities are done on a regular basis).

PHYSICAL ACTIVITY GUIDELINES

It is generally agreed that providing children with a variety and lots of movement experience is important to provide the basis for the development of so-called 'motor skills' (such as those listed in table 14.4). It is also thought that, after the first few years of life, all motor skills are then built on existing ones that the child has already developed. It is important therefore that children are exposed to as wide a variety of motor skills as possible, as soon as possible, to give every child the opportunity to develop these skills. Motor skills, as with cognitive skills, should be taught in a progressive way, but this is often not the case. For instance,

many subjects in the school curriculum are based on a progression of simple information to complex information. Take the example of mathematics, where numeral identification (what is the number), numeral writing (just writing the number), numeral value identification (how much each number is worth), addition, subtraction, multiplication and division are typically taught in this sequence as each area is based on the ones before. Taking part in sports and games activities is a similar concept, however these subjects are not always taught in sequence and progressively as are other subjects. It is important though that they are taught in this way, as all sports are made up of individual locomotor, balance and manipulative skills (see table 14.4) that blend together to make up the complex movement patterns that are seen in sports and games activities. When supervising activities with children, it is important to be aware of the great variety of motor skills that are available and to try to incorporate them as often as possible into play situations, bearing in mind that they should be taught progressively from simple to more complex skills, only progressing when skills are learned. Fundamental movement is a term that is commonly used to describe the development of motor skills in young children.

Care must be taken by those supervising children's activities however, as child development is very individual in that all children progress at different rates and at different ages. In general, though, there are typical age ranges at which children are able to perform certain motor skills. Even though this is a complex subject, table 14.5 gives a very simple guide to the typical motor skills that are associated with certain age ranges.

Table 14.4	Typical motor skills	
Locomotor skills	**Manipulative skills**	**Balance skills**
Walking and running	Throwing and bouncing	Bending and twisting
Jumping, hopping and bounding	Catching and volleying	Stretching and reaching
Galloping and skipping	Striking and kicking	Turning and swaying
Sliding and leaping	Rolling and kicking	Swinging, squatting, pushing and pulling

Table 14.5	Typical age ranges of performed motor skills
Typical age range	**Associated motor skill**
18 months	Climb up not down; walk (forward and back)
18 months–2 years	Gallop (mimic a horse)
2 years	Jump on the spot with both feet
2 years	Roll and kick a ball
3 years	Balance on one foot (static)
3 years	Throw (underarm); hop and skip
4 years	Balance on one foot (longer periods)
4 years	Throw (over arm)

There are many publications relating to guidelines for children and physical activity, however many of these guidelines tend to be broken down into age ranges. This is usually because the difference between the age ranges can be quite dramatic in terms of the type, frequency, intensity and duration of the associated activities. Even though many of the guidelines are slightly different and there is no particular guideline that is generally adopted across the country, most guidelines agree upon an accumulation of at least 30 minutes of moderate to vigorous physical activity on most and preferably all days of the week. All guidelines do agree, however, that this target of 30 minutes can be accumulated in short bouts, such as three 10-minute sessions, or done in one 30-minute session. A slightly different example of physical activity guidelines are those published by the National Association for Sport and Physical Education (NASPE). The guidelines related to the age range 3–5 years are as follows.

1 All children should accumulate at least 60 minutes daily of structured physical activity.

2 Children should engage in at least 60 minutes and up to several hours per day of unstructured physical activity, and should not be sedentary for more than 60 minutes at a time, except when sleeping.

3 They should be given the opportunity to develop competence in movement skills that are considered to be the building blocks for more complex movement tasks.

4   Children should have regular access to indoor and outdoor areas that meet or exceed recommended safety standards of performing large muscle activities.

5   Individuals responsible for the well-being of a pre-school child should be aware of the importance of physical activity and facilitate the child's movement skills.

For children older than the age of 5, however, many of the published guidelines differ greatly compared to those for children under the age of 5. Because of the structure of health and fitness in

Table 14.6	Physical activity guidelines for older children	
	Aerobic training	**Strength training**
Mode	• Any kind of activity that includes weight bearing	• Body weight and bands may be required before progressing to weights
Intensity	• Moderate to vigorous intensity • Choose activities that are intermittent in nature • Emphasise active play rather than exercise for younger children	• Use 8–15 RM • Overload by increasing repetitions then intensity
Duration	• 20–30 minutes per session • 30–60 for overweight and obese	• Perform 1 or 2 sets of 8–10 different exercises • 1–2 minutes' rest between exercises
Frequency	• At least 3 days per week • 6–7 days for overweight and obese	• 2 sessions per week • Encourage other forms of exercise
Precautions	• Be aware of children overheating quickly	• Balance upper and lower body • Overload by increasing repetitions then intensity • Avoid muscular fatigue

General precautions
• All activities should be supervised.
• Learn technique before strength.
• Perform full-range multi-joint exercises if possible.
• Avoid any ballistic movements.
• Perform extended warm-ups/cool-downs.
• Avoid mismatching sizes when pairing/grouping children together.
• If the temperature exceeds 30°C, children should not exercise for longer than 20 minutes, and should be well hydrated before, during and after activities.
• If the temperature exceeds 38°C (100°F), children should not exercise outside.
• It is important for children (and adults) to drink water before, during and after any activity.

this country, the guidelines from the American College of Sports Medicine (ACSM) may be more appropriate, and tend to be widely adopted across the UK. With respect to intensity, duration and frequency of physical activity, table 14.6 gives an overview of the ACSM's physical activity guidelines for children over the age of 5.

It is interesting to know that according to the DH (2004), 1 hour of physical activity each day may not be enough to prevent the current rising obesity trends that can be seen in children. Having said that, 1 hour per day of physical activity may have important health benefits with respect to other diseases. The DH recommends, therefore, that children and young people should achieve a total of at least 60 minutes of at least moderate-intensity physical activity each day. It also recommends that at least twice a week this should include activities to improve bone health, muscle strength and flexibility. The description of moderate intensity that was stated by the DH was 'equivalent to brisk walking, which might leave the participant feeling warm and slightly out of breath'. As with adults, it is often difficult to know at what intensity children are exercising during physical activities. One method that has been developed to help with this is the modified version of the Borg rating of perceived exertion (RPE) scale for children (see table 14.7). As with adults, the scale is shown to children during the activities they are doing and they are asked to say at what level they think they are exercising. The response from the child should help the supervisor to estimate what level they have reached.

Table 14.7	Adapted modified version of Borg's RPE scale for children
Intensity	Explanation
0 rest	How you feel when sitting or resting
1 easy	Light walking; not sweating
2 pretty hard	Playing in the playground and just starting to sweat
3 harder	Playing hard and sweating
4 hard	Running around hard and sweating a lot
5 maximal	Hardest you have ever worked; ready to collapse

RECOMMENDED READING

Ainsworth, B.E., Haskell, W.L., Leon, A.S., Jacobs, D.R., Montoye, H.J., Sallis, J.F. & Paffenbarger, R.S. (1993) Compendium of physical activities: Classification of energy costs of human physical activities. *Medicine and Science in Sports and Exercise*, 25: 71–80

American College of Sports Medicine (2009) *ACSM's guidelines for exercise testing and prescription* (8th edn). London: Lippincott Williams & Wilkins

American Diabetes Association (2000) Type 2 diabetes in children and adolescents. *Pediatrics*, 105: 671–680

Åstrand, P.O., Rodahl, K., Dahl, H.A. & Strømme, S.B. (2003) *Textbook of work physiology: Physiological bases of exercise* (4th edn). Champaign, IL: Human Kinetics

Bao, W., Srinivasan, S.R., Valdez, R., Greenlund, K.J., Wattigney, W.A. & Berenson, G.S. (1997) Longitudinal changes in cardiovascular risk from childhood to young adulthood in offspring of parents with coronary artery disease. *Journal of the American Medical Association*, 278: 1749–1754

Berenson, G.S., Srinivasan, S.R., Bao, W., Newman, W.P., Tracy, R.E. & Wattigney, W.A. (1998) Association between multiple cardiovascular risk factors and atherosclerosis in children and young adults. *New England Journal of Medicine*, 98(338): 1650–1656

BHF National Centre for Physical Activity and Health (2010) *Cost of physical inactivity fact sheet*. Loughborough: British Heart Foundation National Centre for Physical Activity and Health

Biddle, S.J.H., Gorely, T. & Stensel, D.J. (2004) Health-enhancing physical activity and sedentary behaviour in children and adolescents. *Journal of Sport Science*, 22: 679–701

Boreham, C. & Riddoch, C.J. (2001) The physical activity, fitness and health of children. *Journal of Sports Sciences*, 19: 915–929

Cavill, N., Biddle, S. & Sallis, J.F. (2001) Health enhancing physical activity for young people: Statement of the United Kingdom Expert Consensus Conference. *Pediatric Exercise Science*, 13:12–25

Department of Health (2004) *At least 5 a week: Evidence on the impact of physical activity and its relationship to health*. London: Department of Health Publications

Department of Health (2005) *Choosing health, choosing activity. A physical activity action plan*. London: Department of Health Publications

Foresight (2007) *Tackling obesities. Future choices*. London: Foresight

Fox, K.R. (2000) The effects of exercise on self-perceptions and self-esteem. In: Biddle, S.J.H., Fox, K.R. & Boutcher, S.H. (eds) *Physical activity and psychological well-being*. London: Routledge

Freedman, D.S., Dietz, W.H., Srinivasan, S.R. & Berenson, G.S. (1999) The relation of overweight to cardiovascular risk factors among children and adolescents: The Bogalusa Heart Study. *Pediatrics*, 103: 1175–1182

Freedson, P.S. (1991) Electronic motion sensors and heart rate as a measure of physical activity in children. *Journal of School Health*, 61: 220–223

Goran, M.I., Gower, B.A., Nagy, T.R. & Johnson, R. (1998) Developmental changes in energy expenditure and physical activity in children: Evidence for a decline in physical activity in girls prior to puberty. *Pediatrics*, 101: 887–891

Gortmaker, S.L., Must, A., Perrin, J.M., Sobol, A.M. & Dietz, W.H. (1993) Social and economic consequences in adolescence and young adulthood. *New England Journal of Medicine*, 329: 1008–1012

Gruber, J.J. (1986) Physical activity and self-esteem development in children: A meta-analysis. *American Academy of Physical Education Papers*, 19: 330–348

Guthold, R., Cowan, M.J., Autenrieth, C.S., Kann, L. & Riley, L.M. (2010) Physical activity and sedentary behaviour among schoolchildren: A 34-country comparison. *Journal of Pediatrics*, 157(1): 43–49

Hammer, L., Kraemer, H., Wilson, D.M., Ritter, P.L. & Dornbusch, S.M. (1991) Standardised percentile curves of body-mass index for children and adolescents. *American Journal of Diseases of Children*, 145: 259–263

Harsha, D.W. (1995) The benefits of physical activity in childhood. *American Journal of Medicine and Science*, 310(S1): S109–S113

Janz, K.F. (1994) Validation of the CSA accelerometer for assessing children's physical activity. *Medicine and Science in Sports and Exercise*, 26: 369–375

Klesges, R.C., Shelton, M.L. & Klesges, L.M. (1993) Effects of television on metabolic rate: Potential implications for childhood obesity. *Paediatrics*, 91: 281–286

McCurdy, L.E., Winterbottom, K.E., Mehta, S.S. & Roberts, J.R. (2010) Using nature and outdoor activity to improve children's health. *American Journal of Preventative Medicine*, 40(5): 102–117

McGill, H.C., McMahan, C.A., Zieske, A.W., Tracy, R.E., Malcom, G.T., Herderick, E.E. & Strong, J.P. (2000) Association of coronary heart disease risk factors with microscopic qualities of coronary atherosclerosis in youth. *Circulation*, 102: 374–379

McKenzie, T.L., Sallis, J.F., Elder, J.P., Berry, C.C., Hoy, P.L., Nader, P.R., Zive, M.M. & Broyles, S.L. (1997) Physical activity levels and prompts in young children at recess: A two year study of a bi-ethnic sample. *Research Quarterly in Exercise and Sport*, 68: 195–202

Mossberg, H.O. (1989) 40 year follow up of overweight children. *Lancet*, 2: 491–493

Must, A., Jacques, P.F., Dallal, G.E., Bajema, C.J. & Dietz, W.H. (1992) Long term morbidity and mortality of overweight adolescents. A follow-up of the Harvard Growth Study. *New England Journal of Medicine*, 327: 1350–1355

Mutrie, N. & Parfitt, G. (1998) Physical activity and its links with mental, social and moral health in young people. In: Biddle, S., Sallis, J. & Cavill, N. (eds) *Young and active? Young people and health-enhancing physical activity: Evidence and implications*. London: Health Education Authority

NHS Information Centre for Health and Social Care (2009) *Health Survey for England 2008: Physical activity and fitness*. Leeds: NHS Information Centre for Health and Social Care

Nieto, F.J., Szklo, M. & Comstock, G.W. (1992) Childhood weight and growth rate as predictors of adult mortality. *American Journal of Epidemiology*, 136: 201–213

Pellegrini, A.D. & Smith, P.K. (1998) Physical activity play: The nature and function of a neglected aspect of play. *Child Development*, 69: 577–598

Pinhas-Hamiel, O., Dolan, L.M., Daniels, S.R., Standiford, D., Khoury, P.R. & Zeitler, P. (1996) Increased incidence of non-insulin dependent diabetes mellitus among adolescents. *Journal of Pediatrics*, 128: 608–615

Reich, A., Muller, G., Gelbrich, G., Deutscher, K., Godicke, R. & Kiess, W. (2003) Obesity and blood pressure – results from the examination of 2365 schoolchildren in Germany. *International Journal of Obesity*, 27: 1459–1464

Reilly, J.J. (2010) Low levels of objectively measured physical activity in preschoolers in childcare. *Medicine and Science in Sports and Exercise*, 42(3): 502–507

Riddoch, C., Savage, J.M., Murphy, N., Cran, G.W. & Boreham, C. (1991) Long-term health implications of fitness and physical activity patterns. *Archives of Diseases in Children*, 66: 1426–1433

Riddoch, C.J. (1998) Relationships between physical activity and health in young people. In: Biddle, S., Sallis, J. & Cavill, N. (eds) Young and active? *Young people and health-enhancing physical activity: Evidence and implications*. London: Health Education Authority, 17–48

Sallis, J.F., McKenzie, T.L., Kolody, B., Lewis, M., Marshall, S. & Rosengard, P. (1999) Effects of health-related physical education on academic achievement: Project SPARK. *Research Quarterly for Exercise and Sport*, 70: 127–134

Saris, W.H.M. (1986) Habitual physical activity in children: Methodology and findings in health and disease. *Medicine and Science in Sports and Exercise*, 18: 253–263

Schwimmer, J.B., Burwinkle, T.M. & Varni, J.W. (2003) Health-related quality of life of severely obese children and adolescents. *Journal of the American Medical Association*, 289: 1813–1819

Sibley, B.A. & Etnier, J.L. (2003) The relationship between physical activity and cognition in children: A meta-analysis. *Pediatric Exercise Science*, 15: 243–256

Sinaiko, A.R., Donahue, R.P., Jacobs, D.R. & Prineas, R.J. (1999) Relation of weight and rate of increase of weight during childhood and adolescence and body size, blood pressure, fasting insulin and lipids in young adults. The Minneapolis Children's Blood Pressure Study. *Circulation*, 99: 1471–1476

Troiano, R.P. & Flegal, K.M. (1998) Overweight children and adolescents: Description, epidemiology and demographics. *Pediatrics*, 101: 497–504

Twisk, J. (2001) Physical activity guidelines for children and adolescents. A critical review. *Sports Medicine*, 31: 617–627

Twisk, J., Kemper, H.C., van Mechelen, W. & Post, G.B. (1997) Tracking of risk factors for coronary heart disease over a 14-year period: A comparison between lifestyle and biologic risk factors with data from the Amsterdam Growth and Health Study. *American Journal of Epidemiology*, 145: 888–898

Wedderkopp, N., Froberg, K., Hansen, H.S., Riddoch, C. & Andersen, L.B. (2003) Cardiovascular risk factors cluster in children and adolescents with low physical fitness: The European Youth Heart Study (EYHS). *Pediatric Exercise Science*, 15: 419–427

Welk, G.J., Corbin, C.B. & Dale, D. (2000) Measurement issues in the assessment of physical activity in children. *Research Quarterly in Exercise and Sport*, 71: 59–73

World Health Organization (2004) *Young people's health in context. Health Behaviour in School-aged Children (HBSC) study. International report from the 2001/2002 survey*. Copenhagen: WHO Press

USEFUL WEBSITES

American Diabetes Association – www.diabetes.org
British Heart Foundation – www.bhf.org.uk
Department of Health – www.dh.gov.uk
NHS Information Centre for Health and Social Care – www.ic.nhs.uk
World Health Organization – www.who.int/en

OLDER ADULTS 15

15

KEYPOINTS

- The size of the older population is continually increasing, with the amount of people aged 50 years and over rising every year.
- In 2009 there were around 17.7 million people living in England who were aged 50 and over, however by 2029 this will have risen to almost 23 million.
- In the same year there were approximately 9.7 million people aged 65 and older in the UK, and by 2020 one in five of those living in the UK will be aged 65 years or over.
- In 2009 there were around 2.4 million people aged 80 and over living in the UK. By 2029 it is estimated that this figure will have risen to around 4.3 million.
- In 2009 there were approximately 10,200 people aged 100 years and over living in the UK; this figure is expected to rise to a staggering 40,500 by 2028.
- Regular activities of daily living are particularly important for older people, to help encourage independent living.
- Muscular strength and power can be improved, which is important for tasks of daily living such as walking or getting up from a chair.
- Physical activity has been found to be helpful in reducing the incidence of falls.
- Physical activity can help improve the emotional and mental well-being of older people. It is associated with reduced risk of developing depressive symptoms.
- Physical activity can improve some aspects of cognitive function, which are important to tasks of daily living.

WHAT IS IT?

According to the Department of Health (2001) there are three distinct groups of older people.

These are:

1 Entering old age – people who have completed their career in paid employment and/or child

rearing; this is a socially constructed definition of old age and could include people as young as 50; those who fall within this group tend to be active.

2 Transitional phase – a group of older people in transition between healthy, active life and frailty; these people are often in their seventh or eighth decade.

3 Frail older people – those who are vulnerable as a result of health problems, social care needs or a combination of both.

There are considerable physiological changes to the body as the individual gets older. All changes occur at a different rate both within an individual and between individuals, but some of these changes can be slowed down by lifestyle and exercise modification. The physiological process of growing old has often been associated with disease and disability. For this reason, many people think that old age will result in problems such as pain, discomfort, illness, disease, sickness and decreased mobility, and that they will need to

depend on help from friends and family more than they might be used to.

PREVALENCE

The size of the older population is continually increasing, with the amount of people aged 50 and over rising every year. According to the Audit Commission (2008), England's population is ageing and the trend is accelerating. The Commission suggests that the number of older people will increase rapidly in the next 20 years. In 2009 there were around 17.7 million people living in England who were aged 50 years and over, however by 2029 this figure will have risen to almost 23 million people (see fig 15.1). Putting this in percentage terms means that the proportion of the population that is aged 50 or over is also increasing. For example, in 2009, about 34% of people living in England were aged 50 or over, but this figure is expected to rise by about 5% to 39% by 2029.

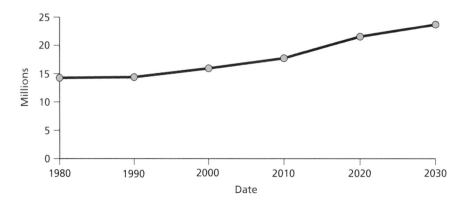

Figure 15.1 Number of people over the age of 50 in England (forecast to 2030)

AGE RANGES IN THE UK

According to the National Institute for Health and Clinical Excellence (NICE) in 2008, there were approximately 9.7 million people aged 65 years or older in the UK (this is almost one in seven) and, by 2020, one in five of those living in the UK will be aged 65 years or older. The number of people aged 80 years and over is also growing rapidly, as with the other age ranges (see fig 15.2). It was estimated that in 2009 there were around 2.4 million people aged 80 years and over living in the UK. By 2029, it is estimated that this figure will have risen to around 4.3 million (almost double). Those people who are 100 years or older (known as centenarians) are the fastest increasing age range of the population. In 2009 there were approximately 10,200 people aged 100 years and over living in the UK, but this figure is expected to rise to a staggering 40,500 by 2028 (almost four times the amount).

It is difficult to say that the growing numbers are as a result of one particular factor as there are many things that might have led to this situation. Such things as declining fertility, which leads to fewer young people, declining mortality rates (deaths) and greater life expectancy as a result of better health care are only some of the factors that may be involved. Regardless of why the numbers are increasing, it is well known that those who live into later life can be affected by such things as physical health, financial security, geographical location, and access to support and services. Also, according to the UK Inquiry into Mental Health and Well-being in Later Life (2006), 40% of older people attending GP surgeries, and 60% of those living in residential institutions, were reported to have 'poor mental health'. Despite better health care provision and increases in wealth over the last 50 years, there is a real danger that the forecast for a massive increase in numbers of older people in the UK could put a massive strain on the health care system such that it might seriously affect the provision capability.

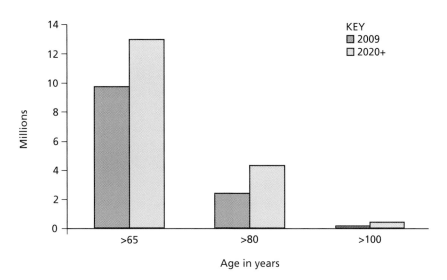

Figure 15.2 Number of people in the UK by age range in 2009 compared to 2020

ASSOCIATED CHANGES

As we get older it is inevitable that we will succumb to both physiological and psychological changes. This process is simply known as ageing. These changes affect people at different stages of their lives and, unfortunately, some people suffer many of the changes whereas others suffer very little change. Table 15.1 briefly describes a range of potential changes.

As can be seen in table 15.1, most functions of the body diminish with age. For example, heart rate slows down by approximately one beat per year from birth. The heart can also become weaker as it is a muscle and needs to be kept in good condition like all other muscles. The deterioration in the heart may also be down to the lifestyle of the individual such as if they smoke or drink regularly. This combination (and other factors) reduces blood flow to all muscles, which means that the supply of oxygen is also decreased. Aerobic capacity (VO_2) also declines from early adulthood and can reduce quite substantially in later years, as shown in table 15.2, to the point where by the age of 75 years aerobic capacity can drop to almost half of its original level.

Table 15.1	Effects of ageing
Area affected	**Description**
Heart	The heart muscle can deteriorate, leading to a reduction in the amount of blood the heart can pump; this means that the amount of oxygen delivered to the muscles will be less
Heart rate	The heart rate slows down after about age 40–50 years, also reducing the oxygen-carrying capacity
Lung function	Vital capacity and forced expiratory volume (see chapter 4) decrease due to several factors, such as breathing muscles becoming weaker and alveoli in the lungs losing elasticity
VO_2 max	Aerobic fitness and respiratory (heart and lungs) function decreases because of the heart and lung changes described above
Flexibility	Muscles lose elasticity; joints become stiff, with a reduction in synovial fluid; cartilage becomes harder (calcifies)
Strength	Decrease in muscle size, motor nerves, mitochondria (where energy is produced) and capillaries
Fat	Increase in adipose (fat tissue) and loss of lean tissue
Brain cells	Brain cells die faster than they are replaced
Senses	Hearing, taste, smell and vision deteriorate, but only about 10% loss
Bones	Bone mineral density decreases, leading to disorders such as spondylosis (narrowing of the spinal canal), osteoporosis (see chapter 9) and postural problems
Blood pressure	Increases with age, mainly due to the hardening of arteries and fatty deposits within them

Table 15.2	Changes in VO₂max among normally active men	
Age (years)	**VO₂max (ml/kg/min)**	**% change from 25 years (approx.)**
25	48	N/A
35	43	10
45	39	18
52	38	20
63	34	29
75	25	48

Source: Adapted from various sources

In relation to physiological and psychological changes, the effects of ageing can be broken down into several areas for better explanation.

CARDIOVASCULAR EFFECTS OF AGEING

The amount of times the heart beats every minute is known simply as the 'heart rate'. The highest possible heart rate a person can achieve is known as 'maximum heart rate'. As a general assumption, maximum heart rate reduces by one beat every year. As the heart is a type of muscle (known as cardiac muscle) it is like any other muscle in that it can weaken if it is not strengthened as much as it should be. The main role of the heart is to pump blood around the body and one of the reasons for this is to provide oxygen to the muscles so that they can do work (contract). If the heart becomes weaker as a result of more sedentary behaviour and is also slower due to age, then the amount of blood that it can pump out becomes less. The amount of blood pumped out of the heart every beat is called 'stroke volume' (SV), and the amount pumped every minute is known as 'cardiac output' (CO).

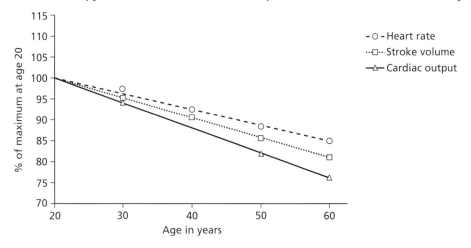

Figure 15.3 Effects of age on heart rate, stroke volume and cardiac output

This can be seen in fig 15.3, which shows how heart rate, stroke volume and cardiac output all decrease in percentage terms, assuming that the maximum capability was around the age of 20 years.

MUSCULAR EFFECTS OF AGEING

The heart is not the only muscle in the body that can weaken with age, as a reduction in muscular strength is also evident within the older population. This can have a negative effect on the daily lives of older people in that they will not be able, or will find it difficult, to perform tasks they once found relatively easy. The loss of muscle mass that occurs as we get older (known as sarcopenia) is one of the main causes of weakness and lack of mobility. Certain types of physical activity can help to slow down the loss of muscle mass, but it cannot stop or reverse the process. Even though the cause of muscle mass loss is not fully understood, it is quite clear that ageing is the main cause and according to studies such as that by Roubenoff and Hughes (2000), inactivity can speed up this process. Many studies over the years have investigated the loss not only of muscular strength but of muscular power as well, because many daily activities (such as getting out of a chair) need muscular power rather than muscular strength alone. For example, investigations by Skelton *et al.* (1995) and Bassey *et al.* (1992) showed that the rate of fall of muscle power was 3.5% per year compared to the rate of fall of muscle strength, which was 1–2% per year. It is important to understand that physical activity needs to continue into old age as, according to studies such as that by Benvenuti *et al.* (2000), physical activity levels up to middle age have no affect on muscle strength in old age. Another problem is that when older people stop doing regular physical activity, the loss of muscle mass and strength occurs faster than it does during youth and middle age. This is a huge problem as loss of muscle strength can increase the risk of osteoporosis and falls, which in turn increases the risk of bone fracture and, as shown in studies such as that by Chu *et al.* (1999), muscle weakness in the legs is linked to the number of falls.

FLEXIBILITY EFFECTS OF AGEING

Not only do muscles lose strength, they also lose elasticity, which means flexibility can be lost too. Flexibility is further affected by the cartilage surrounding joints calcifying, which leads to a decrease in the range of motion at the joint. Because of the loss of muscle strength (and muscle mass) and reduction in flexibility, older people tend not to be as active as they once were, which leads to an increase of adipose tissue and hence fat percentage.

BONE STRENGTH EFFECTS OF AGEING

A reduction in bone strength (due to a decrease in bone mineral density) is a major ageing change that can result in disorders such as osteoporosis and postural problems that are common among elderly people. Loss of bone over the years (known as osteoporosis – see chapter 9) can substantially increase the risk of fractures from falls, which is why it is crucial that regular physical activity is maintained in order to help slow down bone loss and prevent falls. Even though bone strength does not continue to increase once adulthood has arrived (although it is thought that some gain is still possible), it is important to slow down the rate of bone loss. Physical activity, especially strength training, can be of benefit for all ages, although old bone responds more slowly than young bone.

Table 15.3	Common ADL and IADL	
Activities of daily living (ADL)	**Instrumental activities of daily living (IADL)**
Bathing	Cooking
Eating	Shopping
Dressing	Managing money
Toilet duties	Using the telephone
Getting around	Doing housework
	Taking medication

PSYCHOLOGICAL EFFECTS OF AGEING

In relation to psychological changes, older people lose brain cells faster than they are replaced. Senses such as hearing, taste, smell and vision also tend to decrease with age, however these senses tend to deteriorate only up to about a 10% loss. Also, as people get older, they are at increased risk of suffering from conditions such as dementia and Alzheimer's disease.

FUNCTION FOR DAILY LIVING

When talking about the elderly, it is quite common for research to talk in terms of activities of daily living (ADL) and instrumental activities of daily living (IADL) (see table 15.3). It is not surprising to know that the ability to perform ADL and IADL decreases with age. Generally speaking, more than one-third of the UK elderly population will have ADL or IADL problems resulting from chronic health conditions such as arthritis, heart disease and diabetes.

DIAGNOSIS

MUSCULAR STRENGTH AND ENDURANCE

Testing for muscular strength or endurance with older adult groups is quite different from that used with other groups. One common method that is often used (which is really a test of lower body muscle function) is the chair sit-to-stand test (see overleaf). There are a few variations of this test, which differ in the number of the repetitions that subjects are required to perform, including the 30-second test developed by Jones and colleagues (2000).

The arm curl test (see Jones *et al.*, 2000) has been designed because upper body strength and endurance is also needed for carrying out many everyday activities such as cleaning, carrying food shopping and gardening. In this test participants curl a standardised weight as many times as possible in a set amount of time while sitting down (see page 187). The American Alliance for Health, Physical Education, Recreation and Dance (AAHPERD) states that the weight to be used in this test is 4 lb (1.81 kg) for women and 8 lb (3.63 kg) for men.

Test box: Chair sit-to-stand (lower body strength and endurance)

Equipment needed

Stopwatch and a straight-back chair (seat height 44 cm) with no arms. The chair should have rubber tips on the bottom of all legs to stop it from sliding back.

1 The chair should be placed against a wall to prevent any movement.
2 Sit as far back as possible in the chair seat with the feet on the floor approximately hip width apart and the back of lower legs away from the chair. Keep knees bent at a 90-degree angle, with arms over the chest.
3 Let the participant practise standing up to make sure the back of their legs are not touching the chair.
4 The participant then stands up and sits back down as many times as possible in 30 seconds.
5 If participants are unable to stand up once without assistance they can use their hands to assist them in rising and returning to the seated position. Be sure to note that hands were used when recording the assessment data.

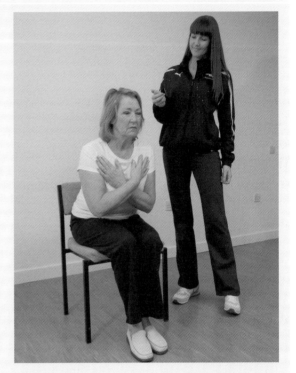

Figure 15.4 Chair sit-to-stand test

Table 15.4	Chair sit-to-stand classification table					
Age range	Men's results			Women's results		
	Below average	Average	Above average	Below average	Average	Above average
60–64	<14	14–19	>19	<12	12–17	>17
65–69	<12	12–18	>18	<11	11–16	>16
70–74	<12	12–17	>17	<10	10–15	>15
75–79	<11	11–17	>17	<10	10–15	>15
80–84	<10	10–15	>15	<9	9–14	>14
85–89	<8	8–14	>14	<8	8–13	>13
90–94	<7	7–12	>12	<4	4–11	>11

Test box: Arm curl (upper body strength and endurance)

Equipment needed

Stopwatch, a straight-back chair (similar to the chair used in the sit-to-stand test) and dumbbells with the selected weight.

1. The aim of this test is to do as many arm curls as possible in 30 seconds on the dominant-arm side (or stronger side).
2. Sit on the chair, holding the weight with palm facing towards the body, arms vertically down beside the chair.
3. Brace the upper arm against the body so that only the lower arm is moving (tester may assist to hold the upper arm steady).
4. Curl the arm up through a full range of motion, gradually turning the palm up (flexion with supination).
5. Lower the arm under control to the starting position.
6. Repeat this action as many times as possible within 30 seconds.

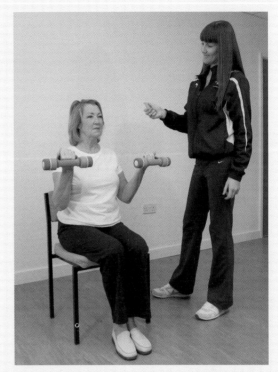

Figure 15.5 Arm curl test

Table 15.5 can be used to classify the participant's score or as a baseline to compare future results.

Table 15.5	Arm curl classification table					
	Men's results			**Women's results**		
Age range	Below average	Average	Above average	Below average	Average	Above average
60–64	<16	16–22	>22	<13	13–19	>19
65–69	<15	15–21	>21	<12	12–18	>18
70–74	<14	14–21	>21	<12	12–17	>17
75–79	<13	13–19	>19	<11	11–17	>17
80–84	<13	13–19	>19	<10	10–16	>16
85–89	<11	11–17	>17	<10	10–15	>15
90–94	<10	10–14	>14	<8	8–13	>13

AEROBIC CAPACITY

One of the other most common activities for older adults is walking, which is why the timed 6-minute walk test was designed to assesses the maximum distance walked in 6 minutes along a rectangular course (Rikli and Jones, 2001).

FLEXIBILITY

The ability to carry out normal everyday functions is absolutely crucial for older people. Flexibility, therefore, is a major component of fitness for this age group. The term flexibility is usually associated with the range of motion around joints in the body. One type of flexibility testing, known as goniometry, is a specific technique where the angle of each joint (or specific joints being measured depending on the requirements of the individual) is measured. The results are then compared against data tables for normal ranges of motion. This type of testing is normally carried out by clinically trained and experienced individuals, therefore simpler methods such as flexion-extension measurements are often used.

One of the most common tests used for hamstring flexibility (it is also a measure of back flexibility) in older adults is the sit-and-reach test (see page 190). There are several variations of this test, such as the modified seated sit-and-reach test

---

Test box: 6-minute walk test (aerobic capacity)

Equipment needed
Tape measure, cones, stopwatch, chairs.

For this test, a flat 50 m rectangular course (20m x 5 m) is marked out in 5 m segments with marker cones as shown below. Make sure chairs are placed at certain points within the course for resting purposes should participants need it.

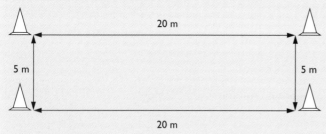

1   Participants line up at a particular starting point (choose one of the cones).
2   Participants are instructed to walk as fast as is comfortable for them, without running, around the course, covering as much distance as possible within the 6-minute time limit.
3   At the end of the test, subjects are told to stop where they are and their distance is measured to the nearest metre.

Rather than have a classification for this particular test, just record the distance and use this as a baseline so that further tests can be compared for improvement.

Test box: Flexibility (back flexion, lateral flexion and extension)

Equipment needed
Tape measure.

Lumbar flexion (see fig 15.6a)
1   Stand upright on the floor with the arms hanging at the side of the body.
2   Bend forward from the trunk as far as possible, keeping the legs straight, and reach towards the floor.
3   The tester measures the vertical distance from the tips of the fingers to the floor.

Lumbar extension (see fig 15.6b)
1   Stand upright on the floor with the arms hanging by the side.
2   Bend backwards from the trunk as far as possible, keeping the legs straight.
3   With the palms facing forwards, keep the arms straight and in a vertical line to the floor.
4   Measure the vertical distance between the tips of the fingers and the floor.

Lateral lumbar flexion (see fig 15.6c)
1   Stand upright on the floor with the arms hanging at the side of the body and the palms facing inwards. The feet should be hip distance apart.
2   Bend sideways from the trunk as far as possible, keeping the legs straight, and reach towards the floor with a straight arm.
3   The tester measures the vertical distance from the tips of the fingers to the floor.

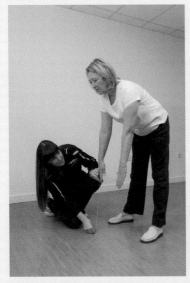 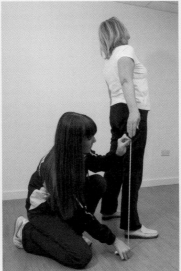 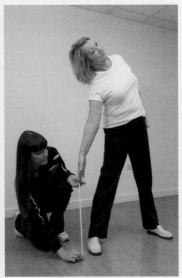

Figure 15.6a Lumbar flexion   **Figure 15.6b** Lumbar extension   **Figure 15.6c** Lat lumbar flexion

Test box: Sit-and-reach (hamstring and upper back flexibility)

Equipment needed
A sit-and-reach box or a bench and ruler.

Testing method
1 Allow the participant to fully warm up and stretch before the test.
2 The participant's legs should be fully extended with the feet (no shoes) flat against the vertical surface of the box.
3 With one hand placed over the other (palms down, arms straight, fingers outstretched), the participant should lean forwards as far as possible, sliding his or her hand along the ruler of the sit-and-reach box.
4 The maximal distance the fingers reach is recorded.
5 The subject must keep their hands parallel and should not lead with one hand.

6 Make several attempts and record the best score.

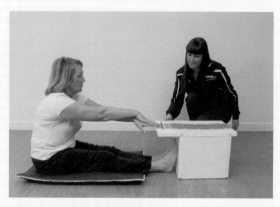

Figure 15.7 Sit-and-reach test

Table 15.6 can be used to classify the participant's score or as a baseline to compare future results.

Table 15.6	Sit-and-reach classification table				
Gender	Excellent	Above average	Average	Below average	Poor
Male	≥18 cm	6–17 cm	0–5 cm	-8 to -1 cm	≤-9 cm
Female	≥21 cm	11–20 cm	1–10 cm	-7 to 0 cm	≤-8 cm

and the chair sit-and-reach test. If participants cannot hold a seated position on the floor then they should use the adapted seated sit-and-reach test. In both variations of the test the subjects should hold their final position for 2 seconds and the distance to the nearest centimetre is recorded.

The chair sit-and-reach test (see page 191) is a variation of the traditional sit-and-reach test, and is also a measure of hamstring and upper back flexibility. This test is useful for those individuals who might find it difficult to do the standard floor sit-and-reach test.

BALANCE
Static balance tests such as the stork stand test (see page 192) are a common measure of balance for all populations. These tests can also be adapted to measure the ability of the elderly to balance under certain conditions, such as reduced base support with the eyes open or closed. For example: feet

Test box: Chair sit-and-reach (hamstring and upper back flexibility)

Equipment needed
Ruler, straight back or folding chair (about 17 in/ 44 cm high).

1 Sit on the edge of a chair with one foot flat on the floor. The other leg is extended forward with the knee straight, heel on the floor (ankle bent at 90°).
2 Place one hand on top of the other, with tips of the middle fingers even.
3 Inhale, then when exhaling reach forwards slowly towards the toes. Keep the back straight and head up, and hold the reach for 2 seconds.
4 Measure the distance between the fingertips and the toes to the nearest cm.
5 If the fingertips touch the toes then the score is zero. If they do not touch, measure the distance between the fingers and the toes (a negative score), if they overlap, measure by how much (a positive score). The score is recorded to the nearest ½ in or 1 cm as the distance reached – either a negative or positive score.

6 Record which leg was used for measurement.

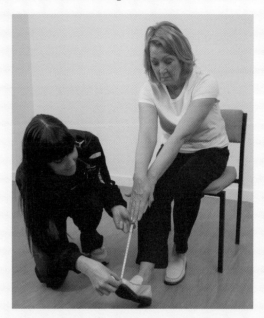

Figure 15.8 Chair sit-and-reach test

Table 15.7 can be used to classify the participant's score or as a baseline to compare future results.

Table 15.7	Chair sit-and-reach classification table					
	Men's results			**Women's results**		
Age range	**Below average**	**Average**	**Above average**	**Below average**	**Average**	**Above average**
60–64	<−5	−5 to 8	>8	<−1	−1 to 10	>10
65–69	<−6	−6 to 6	>6	<−1	−1 to 9	>9
70–74	<−7	−7 to 5	>5	<−2	−2 to 8	>8
75–79	<−8	−8 to 4	>4	<−3	−3 to 7	>7
80–84	<−11	−11 to 3	>3	<−4	−4 to 6	>6
85–89	<−11	−11 to 1	>1	<−5	−5 to 5	>5
90–94	<−13	−13 to 1	>1	<9	−9 to 2	>2

touching, side by side; one foot moved half a length forward; one foot in front of the other, heel to toe. The test usually measures the maximum amount of time for which the participant can hold the stance, however the test can be stopped after a certain amount of time depending on the participant.

Test box: Stork stand test (static balance)

Equipment needed
Chair, stopwatch.

1 Stand comfortably with both feet on the floor and hands on hips.
2 Lift one leg and place the toes of that foot against the knee of the other leg.
3 On command raise the heel to stand on the toes.
4 The stopwatch is then started and participants are to balance for as long as possible without letting either the heel touch the ground or the other foot move away from the knee. Repeat on the opposite leg.

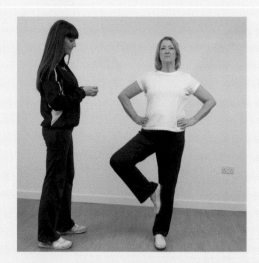

Figure 15.9 Stork stand test

NB: Due to the potential risk of falling associated with this test it is advised not to compare the score against any norm tables, but just to use it as a baseline for each leg to compare against future test scores.

Table 15.8	Typical benefits of exercise and activity for older adults	
Physical benefits	**Psychological benefits**
• Controlling high blood pressure	• Improved mental health
• Reduction in blood pressure	• Decreased anxiety
• Reduction in blood lipids	• Increased self-esteem
• Maintenance of arterial flexibility	• Increase in confidence
• Improved motor function	• Improved cognitive function
	• Delayed memory loss

PHYSICAL ACTIVITY BENEFITS

Any form of physical activity in later life is crucial for improving or just maintaining health. It is widely agreed that regular physical activity has many beneficial effects on physical and psychological health (as listed in table 15.8), both of which can help the individual to retain independence further into later life.

AEROBIC FITNESS BENEFITS

It is a misconception that fitness levels cannot be improved in later life. Aerobic capacity can be improved at any age, even if chronic breathing problems are present. Aerobic-type activity is recommended for older adults regardless of age as long as the starting point is just above the level that each individual is accustomed to.

MUSCULAR STRENGTH AND POWER BENEFITS

There is a general agreement that muscle strength decreases at a rate of about 10% per decade up to as much as 60% total loss by the age of 80. Therefore, regular strength training for older adults using external weights or body weight (resistance exercises) should not be underestimated as it has been shown to be highly effective in increasing or just maintaining muscle strength, even into very old age. For example, in an investigation by Narici (2000), older adults exercised for two to three sessions per week with loads greater than 65% of 1 RM (1 RM = the 1 repetition maximum, or the maximum load that can be lifted once only) and showed significant improvements in muscle strength similar to improvements observed in young adults. Just like aerobic fitness, there is a general agreement that muscle strength can be improved at any age by following a progressive resistance training programme. As an indirect result of this, bone density and resting metabolism as well as muscle strength can be increased, which will help individuals to perform activities of daily living as described earlier.

FLEXIBILITY BENEFITS

The loss of mobility as a result of a decrease in flexibility can lead to many negative effects, such as deprivation of sleep, decline of functional capacity and decreased organ function. Ideally, all major muscle groups should be stretched on a daily basis but, just like aerobic activities, the starting point of the flexibility exercises should be just above the level to which each individual is accustomed.

BENEFITS TO DEPRESSION

There is an abundance of research to show that physical activity can help improve the emotional and mental well-being of older people. For example, it has been shown on many occasions that physical activity is associated with reduced clinical and non-clinical depression among older people, and can also help to reduce anxiety and enhance mood (even when there is no improvement in fitness levels). Rehabilitation programmes incorporating physical activity have had positive effects on the emotional functioning and mental health of older people. Possibly one of the main psychological benefits of physical activity in older age groups is related to other conditions that people might have. For example, studies such as those by Kugler *et al.* (1994), Mock *et al.* (1997) and Carrieri-Kohlman *et al.* (1996) have shown that with older people who are cardiac rehabilitation patients, those with chronic obstructive pulmonary disease (COPD), breast cancer patients and osteoarthritic patients, physical activity produces a small to moderate reduction in anxiety and symptoms of depression.

COGNITIVE FUNCTION BENEFITS

One area that is regarded as 'psychological' is that of cognition or cognitive thinking. In simple terms, cognition just means to think. Cognitive functioning can include areas such as speed and accuracy of response, working memory and multiple task processing, which all deteriorate with age and can have a traumatic effect on older people. Research in this area is limited but does show that physical activity can improve at least some of the areas of cognitive function among older people. For example, research such as that by Boutcher (2000) has shown that those people with higher aerobic fitness, and higher levels of activity and sport participation, are better able to manage cognitive tasks. A word of caution is needed here as not all research has found such improvement, as in the work by Biddle and Faulkner (2002) and Etnier *et al.* (1997). However, more recent studies, such as that by Colcombe and Kramer (2003), have shown that exercise training resulted in benefits in processes such as short-term memory, decision making and quick thinking.

BENEFITS TO DEMENTIA AND ALZHEIMER'S DISEASE

As mentioned earlier in this chapter, as people get older they have an increased risk of conditions such as dementia and Alzheimer's disease. Some long-term studies have shown that regular physical activity may be of benefit to these conditions,

which are associated with old age. For example, studies by McDowell (2001), Laurin *et al.* (2001) and Schuit *et al.* (2001) have shown that high levels of physical activity reduce the risk of Alzheimer's disease and dementia. Another interesting aspect can be seen in a study by Yaffe *et al.* (2001) in which women, aged 65 years or older with a greater physical activity level, were less likely to experience a decline in cognitive function during the 6 to 8 years of follow-up as those women with lower fitness levels.

FUNCTION FOR DAILY LIVING BENEFITS

Remaining physically active in older age is essential for helping people to maintain their independence. Activities for daily living are often the most important aspect for older people. Activities such as walking to local shops, attending group meetings and daily outings, which can be done with less reliance on others, are vital for promoting social and community interaction. Even though there is little direct evidence to support this, anecdotally, positive social benefits are often found in physical activity programmes involving older people.

PHYSICAL ACTIVITY GUIDELINES

The aims of a physical activity programme should be to reduce the physical deterioration and social dysfunction of older individuals. Emphasis should be placed on the improvement of ability with respect to the performance of everyday activities, as there are many positive benefits of regular physical activity.

Table 15.9	Physical activity guidelines for sedentary older adults	
	Aerobic training	**Strength training**
Mode	• Walking, cycling and water-based activities are better for those with reduced tolerance for weight bearing	• Body weight and bands may be required before progressing to weights
Intensity	• Work to individual capacity	• Overload by increasing repetitions before intensity
Duration	• 20–30 minutes per session • Increase duration rather than intensity • Slow progression	• Perform 2 to 3 sets of 12–15 RM • 1–2 minutes' rest between exercises
Frequency	• 3–5 days per week	• 2–3 sessions per week • Encourage other forms of exercise
Precautions	• Constantly monitor feedback and use RPE scales	• Avoid muscular fatigue • Balance upper and lower body

General precautions
• Be wary when setting goals as progression is often slow.
• Get feedback relating to muscle soreness, especially if the individual is inexperienced.
• Relaxation is recommended post-exercise.
• Give consideration to any condition the individual may have.

Functional activities are highly recommended as part of an overall activity programme. The list of functional activities, however, can be endless and specific to the needs of the individual. Having said that, there are many common types of movement or activity that can be classed as functional as they relate to everyday life and tasks. Appendix 1 at the end of this chapter gives a selection of such activities that are useful to a variety of older age adults, but predominantly for those that have little background in exercise or have low fitness levels. All of the activities can be done without the use of any equipment. If equipment is available (such as resistance bands or foam cushions), then the range of activities is endless. It is advisable to start with mobilisation exercises first so that joints can be prepared for the activities to follow. Ambulation exercises are those that involve the movement of the body from one place to another in a variety of directions. This may sound straightforward but ask yourself the question 'How often do I practise walking backwards or sideways?' Balance exercises are recommended to be done either on separate occasions or before strength-based exercises, as fatigue from the strength-based exercises could have an effect on the balance exercises.

It is difficult to give guidelines for the frequency, duration, sets and repetitions and so on, as like any other population, older age people will have different levels of ability. For this reason, each exercise should be tried out to establish a baseline level that the individual can cope with and this should be used as the starting point for the programme. Remember, though, that progression will be very slow for this population group.

APPENDIX 1

AMBULATION EXERCISES FOR OLDER AGE PEOPLE

HEEL STANDS AND HEEL WALKS

1. Stand on heels with support (fig 15.10a).
2. Stand on heels without support.
3. Walk along a straight line on heels with support (fig 15.10b).
4. Walk along a straight line on heels without support.

TOE STANDS AND TOE WALKS

1. Stand on toes with support (fig 15.11a).
2. Stand on toes without support.
3. Walk along a straight line on toes with support (fig 15.11b).
4. Walk along a straight line on toes without support.

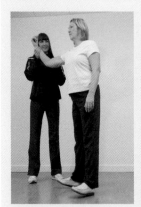

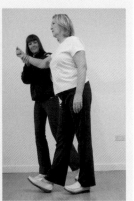

Figure 15.10a Stand on heels with support

Figure 15.10b Walk on heels with support

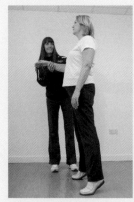

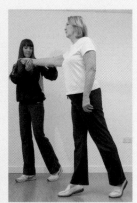

Figure 15.11a Stand on toes with support

Figure 15.11b Walk on toes with support

MULTI-DIRECTION STRAIGHT-LINE WALKING

1 Walk with support in a straight line forwards.
2 Walk without support in a straight line forwards.
3 Walk with support in a straight line backwards (fig 15.12a).
4 Walk without support in a straight line backwards.
5 Walk with support in a straight line sideways (go both ways) (fig 15.12b).
6 Walk without support in a straight line sideways (go both ways).

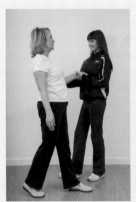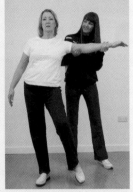

Figure 15.12a Walk backwards with support

Figure 15.12b Walk sideways with support

STEPPING

1 Step up on to a step with the leading leg, touch the step with the other leg and return with support. Change legs (fig 15.13a).
2 Step up on to a step with the new leading leg, touch the step with the other leg and return without support. Change legs.
3 Step up on to a step with one leg then on to the next step with the other, and so on, with support.
4 Step up on to a step with the new leg then on to the next step with the other, and so on, without support.
5 Step down on to a step with the leading leg, touch the step with the other leg and return with support. Change legs (15.13b).
6 Step down on to a step with the new leading leg, touch the step with the other leg and return with support. Change legs.
7 Step down on to a step with one leg then on to the next step with the other, and so on, with support.
8 Step down on to a step with the new leg then on to the next step with the other, and so on, without support.

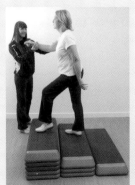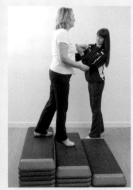

Figure 15.13a Step up, touch, step back

Figure 15.13b Step down, touch step back

MOBILISATION EXERCISES FOR OLDER AGE PEOPLE

SHOULDER MOBILISATION (SITTING OR STANDING)

1   Swing both arms forwards and backwards under control to the end range of motion (alternately or together) (fig 15.14a).
2   Swing both arms out to the side under control to the end range of motion then bring the arms back to cross the front of the body (fig 15.14b).
3   Change the position of the feet if standing (wide stance, narrow stance, split stance).

TRUNK MOBILISATION (SITTING OR STANDING)

1   Put the hands on the hips and rotate the upper body only leading with the elbow. Go in both directions and try not to move the hips (fig 15.15a).
2   Put the hands on the hips and bend forwards with the upper body only, then return to the upright position.
3   Put the hands on the hips and lean to the side with the upper body only and hips firmly in position. Do on the other side (15.15b).

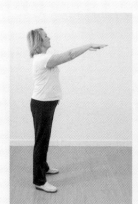
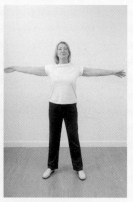

Figure 15.14a Forward arm swing

Figure 15.14b Side arm swing

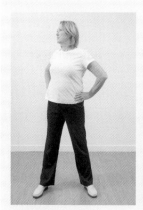
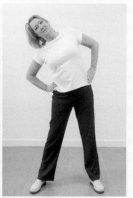

Figure 15.15a Trunk rotation

Figure 15.15b Trunk side flexion

PELVIS MOBILISATION

1 While sitting upright, tilt the pelvis forwards (fig 15.16a) and backwards (fig 15.16b).
2 Lift the left and right buttocks alternately while sitting and pushing the buttocks into the chair.
3 Make circles (in both directions) by pelvic rotation.
4 Repeat steps 1–3 while standing with the knees slightly bent.

FOOT AND ANKLE MOBILISATION (SITTING OR STANDING)

1 Point the foot forwards then pull the foot backwards while keeping the heel on the floor. Change legs (fig 15.17a).
2 Repeat with the heel off the floor.
3 Make circles with the front of the foot while keeping the heel on the floor. Change legs.
4 Repeat with the heel off the floor (fig 15.17b).

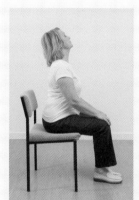

Figure 15.16a
Forward pelvis tilt

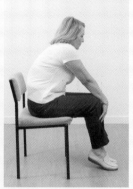

Figure 15.16b
Backward pelvis tilt

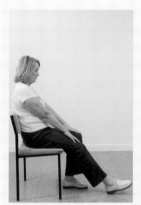

Figure 15.17a Foot point, heel on floor

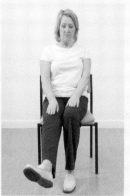

Figure 15.17b Ankle circle, heel off floor

BALANCE EXERCISES FOR OLDER AGE PEOPLE

ONE-LEG STAND

1. Stand on one leg with support.
2. Stand on one leg without support (fig 15.18a).
3. Stand on one leg with support and eyes closed.
4. Stand on one leg without support and eyes closed (have support near).
5. Stand on one leg with support holding an object.
6. Stand on one leg without support holding an object (fig 15.18b).
7. Stand on one leg with support holding an object and eyes closed.
8. Stand on one leg without support holding an object and eyes closed.

BALANCE WALKS

1. Walk very slowly forwards on a straight line with support (fig 15.19a).
2. Walk very slowly forwards on a straight line without support.
3. Walk very slowly forwards on a straight line with support and eyes closed.
4. Walk very slowly forwards on a straight line without support and eyes closed, but make sure someone is very close to steady if needed (fig 15.19b).

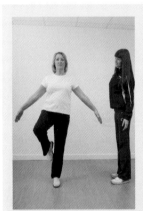

Figure 15.18a One leg stand no support

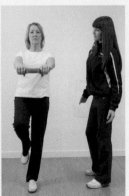

Figure 15.18b One leg, holding object, eyes closed

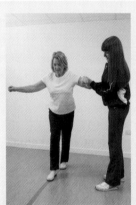

Figure 15.19a Walk forward with support

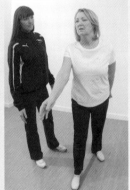

Figure 15.19b Walk with eyes closed without support

STRENGTH-BASED EXERCISES FOR OLDER AGE PEOPLE

CHAIR STAND (USE FIRM CHAIR THAT IS ADJUSTABLE, IF POSSIBLE)

1   From a seated position and with the use of the arms for push-off, come to a standing position with support (fig 15.20a).

2   From a seated position and with the use of the arms for push-off, come to a standing position without support.

3   From a seated position and with no use of the arms for push-off, come to a standing position with support (fig 15.20b).

4   From a seated position and with no use of the arms for push-off, come to a standing position without support.

CHAIR SIT (USE FIRM CHAIR THAT IS ADJUSTABLE, IF POSSIBLE)

1   From a standing position and with the use of the arms to steady, lower slowly to a seated position with support (fig 15.21a).

2   From a standing position and with the use of the arms to steady, lower slowly to a seated position without support.

3   From a standing position and with no use of the arms, lower to a seated position with support (fig 15.21b).

4   From a standing position and with no use of the arms, lower to a seated position without support.

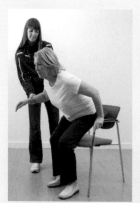
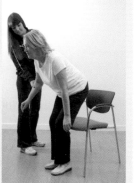

Figure 15.20a Stand up with arms, support

Figure 15.20b Stand up, no arms, support

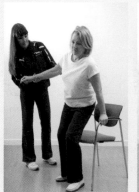
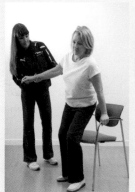

Figure 15.21a Sit down with arms, support

Figure 15.21b Sit down, no arms, support

RECOMMENDED READING

American College of Sports Medicine (2009a) *ACSM's exercise management for persons with chronic diseases and disabilities* (3rd edn). Champaign, IL: Human Kinetics

American College of Sports Medicine (2009b) *ACSM's guidelines for exercise testing and prescription* (8th edn). London: Lippincott Williams & Wilkins

Audit Commission (2004) *Older people. Independence and well-being: The challenge for public services*. London: Audit Commission

Audit Commission (2008) *Don't stop me now. Preparing for an ageing population*. London: Audit Commission

Bassey, E.J., Fiatarone, M.A., O'Neill, E.F., Kelly, M., Evans, W.J. & Lipsitz, L.A. (1992) Leg extensor power and functional performance in very old men and women. *Clinical Science*, 82: 321–327

Benvenuti, E., Bandinelli, S., Di Iorio, A., Gangemi, S., Camici, S. & Lauretani, F. (2000) Relationship between motor behaviour in young/middle age and level of physical activity in late life. Is muscle strength the causal pathway? In: Capodaglio, P. & Narici, M.V. (eds) *Advances in rehabilitation*. Pavia, Italy: PI-ME Press, 17–27

Bernard, M. (2000) *Promoting health in old age: Critical issues in self health care*. Buckingham: Open University Press

Biddle, S. & Faulkner, G. (2002) Psychological and social benefits of physical activity. In: Chan, K.M., Chodzko-Zajko, W., Frontera, W. & Parker, A. (eds) *Active ageing*. Hong Kong: Lippincott Williams & Wilkins Asia Ltd, 89–164

Bouchard, C., Shephard, R.J. & Stephens, T. (1994) *Physical activity, fitness and health*. Champaign, IL: Human Kinetics

Boutcher, S.H. (2000) Cognitive performance, fitness and ageing. In: Biddle, S.J.H., Fox, K.R. & Boutcher, S.H. (eds) *Physical activity and psychological well-being*. London: Routledge, 118–129

Carrieri-Kohlman, V., Gormley, J.M., Douglas, M.K., Paul, S.M. & Stulbarg, M.S. (1996) Exercise training decreases dyspnea and the distress and anxiety associated with it. Monitoring alone may be as effective as coaching. *Chest*, 110: 1526–1535

Chu, L.W., Pei, C.K., Chiu, A., Liu, K., Chu, M.M., Wong, S. & Wong. A. (1999) Risk factors for falls in hospitalized older medical patients. *Journals of Gerontology Series A, Biological Sciences and Medical Sciences*, 54: M38–M43

Colcombe, S. & Kramer, A.F. (2003) Fitness effects on the cognitive function of older adults: A meta-analytic study. *Psychological Science*, 14: 125–130

Department of Health (2001) *National service framework for older people*. London: HMSO

Department of Health (2005a) *Everybody's business: Integrated mental health services for older adults: A service development guide*. London: HMSO

Department of Health (2005b) *Choosing activity: A physical activity action plan*. London: HMSO

Department of Health (2005c) *Securing better mental health as part of active ageing*. London: HMSO

Etnier, J.L., Salazar, W., Landers, D.M., Petruzzello, S.J., Han, M. & Nowell, P. (1997) The influence of physical fitness and exercise upon cognitive functioning: A meta analysis. *Journal of Sport and Exercise Psychology*, 19: 249–277

Faber, M.J., Bosscher, R.J., Chin A Paw, M.J. & van Wieringen, P.C. (2006) Effects of exercise programs on falls and mobility in frail and pre-frail older adults: A multicenter randomized controlled trial. *Archives of Physical Medical Rehabilitation*, 87: 885–896

Finch, H. (1997) *Physical activity 'at our age'. Qualitative research among people over the age of 50*. London: Health Education Authority

Fitzgerald, M.D., Tanaka, H., Tran, Z.V. & Seals, D.R. (1997) Age-related declines in maximal aerobic capacity in regularly exercising vs sedentary women: A meta-analysis. *Journal of Applied Physiology*, 83: 160–165

Frontera, W.R., Hughes, V.A., Lutz, K.J. & Evans, W.J. (1991) A cross-sectional study of muscle strength and mass in 40- to 78-yr-old men and women. *Journal of Applied Physiology*, 71: 644–650

Health Promotion England (2001) *Older people and physical activity*. Physical education factsheet. London: Health Promotion England

Jones, C.J. & Rikli, R.E. (2002) Measuring functional fitness of older adults. *Journal on Active Ageing*, 1: 24–30

Jones, C.J., Rikli, R.E., Max, J. & Noffal, G. (1998) The reliability and validity of a chair sit and reach test as a measure of hamstring flexibility in older adults. *Research Quarterly for Exercise and Sport*, 69: 338–343

Jones, C.J., Rikli, R.E. & Beam, W.C. (2000) A 30-s chair-stand test to measure lower body strength in community-residing older adults. *Journal of Ageing and Physical Activity*, 8: 85

Kugler, J., Seelbach, H. & Kruskemper, G.M. (1994) Effects of rehabilitation exercise programmes on anxiety and depression in coronary patients: A meta-analysis. *British Journal of Clinical Psychology*, 33: 401–410

Latham, N.K., Bennett, D.A., Stretton, C.M. & Anderson, C.S. (2004) Systematic review of progressive resistance strength training in older adults. *Journal of Gerontology Series A Biological Sciences and Medical Sciences*, 59: M48–M61

Laurin, D., Verreault, R., Lindsay, J., MacPherson, K. & Rockwood, K. (2001) Physical activity and risk of cognitive impairment and dementia in elderly persons. *Archives of Neurology*, 58: 498–504

McAuley, E., Kramer, A.F. & Colcombe, S.J. (2004) Cardiovascular function in older adults: A brief review. *Brain, Behavior and Immunity*, 18: 214–220

McDowell, I. (2001) Alzheimer's disease: Insights from epidemiology. *Ageing*, 13: 143–162

Merchant, J., Griffin, B.L. & Charnock, A. (2007) *Sport and physical activity: The role of health promotion.* Basingstoke: Palgrave Macmillan

Mertz, K.J., Lee, D.C., Sui, X., Powell, K.E. & Blair, S.N. (2010) Falls among adults: The association of cardiorespiratory fitness and physical activity with walking related falls. *American Journal of Preventative Medicine*, 39(1): 15–24

Mock, V., Dow, K.H., Meares, C.J., Grimm, P.M., Dienemann, J.A., Haisfield-Wolfe, M.E., Quitasol, W., Mitchell, S., Chakravarthy, A. & Gage, I. (1997) Effects of exercise on fatigue, physical functioning, and emotional distress during radiation therapy for breast cancer. *Oncology Nursing Forum*, 24: 991–1000

Narici, M.V. (2000) Structural and functional adaptations to strength training in the elderly. In: Capodaglio, P. & Narici, M.V. (eds) *Advances in rehabilitation.* Pavia, Italy: PI-ME Press, 55–60

Pendergast, D.R., Fisher, N.M. & Calkins, E. (1993) Cardiovascular, neuromuscular and metabolic alterations with age leading to frailty. *Journal of Gerontology*, 48: 61–67

Rikli, R.E. & Jones, C.J. (1997) Assessing physical performance in independent older adults: Issues and guidelines. *Journal of Ageing and Physical Activity*, 5: 244–261

Rikli, R.E. & Jones, C.J. (2001) *Senior fitness test manual.* Champaign, IL: Human Kinetics

Roubenoff, R. & Hughes, V.A. (2000) Sarcopenia: Current concepts. *Journals of Gerontology Series A, Biological Sciences and Medical Sciences*, 55: M716–M724

Różańska-Kirschke, A., Kocur, P., Wilk, M. & Dylewicz, P. (2006) The Fullerton Fitness Test as an index of fitness in the elderly. *Medical Rehabilitation*, 10(2): 9–16

Schuit, A.J., Feskens, E.J., Launer, L.J. & Kromhout, D. (2001) Physical activity and cognitive decline, the role of the apolipoprotein e4 allele. *Medicine and Science in Sports and Exercise*, 33: 772–777

Skelton, D.A. & McLaughlin, A.W. (1996) Training functional ability in old age. *Physiotherapy*, 82(3): 159–167

Skelton, D.A., Young, A., Greig, C.A. & Malbut, K.E. (1995) Effects of resistance training on strength, power, and selected functional abilities of women aged 75 and older. *Journal of the American Geriatrics Society*, 43: 1081–1087

UK Inquiry into Mental Health and Well-being in late life (2006) *Promoting mental health and well-being in later life.* London: Age Concern and Mental Health Foundation

Yaffe, K., Barnes, D., Nevitt, M., Lui, L.Y. & Covinsky, K. (2001) A prospective study of physical activity and cognitive decline in elderly women: Women who walk. *Archives of Internal Medicine*, 161: 1703–1708

USEFUL WEBSITES

Audit Commission – www.audit-commission.gov.uk
Department of Health – www.dh.gov.uk
Health Education Authority – www.nice.org.uk
www.hea.org.uk
National Institute for Health and Clinical Excellence – www.hea.org.uk

DISABILITY AND INCLUSION 16

WHAT IS IT?

In this chapter there are two terms that need to be understood as they are interrelated in terms of the provision of physical activity for this particular population. It is important therefore that the terms 'disability' and 'inclusion' are first described.

DISABILITY

The term disability can be one of the most controversial and difficult to try to describe. One of the reasons for this is that the definition could be based on various models such as a medical model or a social model. In the case of the medical model, an individual can be born with a so-called disability such as Down's syndrome or cerebral palsy, or they could acquire a disability through an illness, chronic disease or as the result of an injury. Also within the medical model there could be mental health problems such as depression, dementia and schizophrenia, which are commonly thought of as disabilities. However, some definitions refer to a social model of disability: how some people do not 'fit in' and are therefore considered to be disabled. Whatever the accepted definition or model of disability, they can vary widely in terms of type, severity and duration. For example, disabilities can affect a person's ability to walk, see, hear, understand or speak. Because of this extreme variation, it is important to understand that every disability is different and even the same type or category of disability can affect each individual differently. It is better therefore to focus less on the definition of disability and to think in terms of what disabled people can do rather than any restrictions that they might have relating to a particular condition. According to the English Federation of Disability Sport there are between 8 and 12 million people in the UK with some degree of disability or impairment as defined by 'disabled' under the Disability Discrimination Act (DDA). As far as catering for sport or fitness provision is concerned, the Disability Discrimination Act 2005 provides guidance on the acts and regulations relating to this area.

INCLUSION

The use of the term inclusion is becoming more widespread, especially in schools and sports clubs. This particular term simply means to create environments that are accessible, safe and supportive of persons of all ages, gender and

ability. There are many barriers that are experienced by people with disabilities that cannot be seen, such as the negative attitudes of others, lack of knowledge or difficult communication situations. Barriers such as these should never be allowed to exist as there are many simple things that can be done to ensure that all individuals are given the same opportunities to participate in physical activity. Simple solutions, such as providing the necessary adaptive equipment (including accessible fitness, sports or recreation equipment) to allow individuals with disabilities to participate fully, are easy to put in place. It can also help if those delivering sessions know how to use specialised equipment and how to adapt activities for different disabilities.

TERMINOLOGY

People are often confused about what they think is the correct terminology to use when relating to disability. The attempt to be 'politically correct' can often create confusion and embarrassing situations, so it is recommended that, if people are unsure about the terminology to use, simply asking the person with the disability what they would prefer would be the easiest solution. Table 16.1 gives an overview of just some of the current terms that are used in relation to various disabilities. It must be mentioned, however, that these terms can change in their 'political correctness' so it is always recommended to visit the website of the leading body related to each disability for the up-to-date information.

It is an unfortunate fact that, in today's society, there are many misconceptions about individuals with disabilities. Many of these misconceptions are not based on any particular evidence, and it is usually a lack of understanding or ignorance that

Table 16.1	Common terms related to disability
Terms	**Description**
Disability	General term used for a functional limitation that interferes with a person's ability and can be a physical, sensory or mental condition
Non-disabled	This was previously able-bodied
Handicap	A physical or attitudinal constraint imposed upon a person, regardless of whether or not that person has a disability
Hemiplegia	Full or partial paralysis of one side of the body
Paraplegia	Paralysis of the lower half of the body, including the partial or total loss of function of both legs
Quadriplegia	Paralysis of the body involving partial or total loss of function in both arms and legs
Down's syndrome	A chromosome disorder that usually causes a delay in physical, intellectual and language development; usually results in mental retardation; joints can also be unstable due to lax ligaments; 'mongol' is an unacceptable term
Hearing impairment	Refers to partial or total loss of auditory functioning; not referred to as 'the deaf' but use 'people who are deaf'
Speech impairment	Some level of speech problem that causes speaking difficulty
Cerebral palsy	Brain lesions leading to movement and speech problems; not called 'spasticity' any more
Additional needs	Used to be called special needs
Learning disability	A group of neurological conditions (e.g. dyslexia, dysgraphia, dyscalculia) that affect the person's ability to receive, interpret and use information
Mental disability	Psychiatric disability, retardation, learning disability and cognitive impairment
Muscular dystrophy	A condition that affects muscle fibres and causes weakness; often results in the use of a powered wheelchair

Table 16.2	Common misconceptions related to disability	
Misconception		**Reality**
Having a disability means that you are not or cannot be healthy		People with disabilities can achieve good health as they can benefit from healthy activities as much as the general population
Wheelchair use implies that users of wheelchairs are 'wheelchair bound'		A wheelchair, much the same as a bicycle, is just a personal assistive device that helps someone to get around
You shouldn't ask people about their disabilities		Most people with disabilities won't mind answering any questions
People with disabilities always need help		Many people with disabilities are quite independent, but if you want to help then just ask them if they need any

appears to be the main problem. Even as recently as 20 or 30 years ago, there was limited access for the public regarding information related to specific disabilities. Today, however, this is just not the case as the amount of publicity and information that is commonly available is vast and easily accessible. Table 16.2 gives an overview of just some of the most common misconceptions that people have about those with disabilities, and what the reality associated with disability generally is.

WHAT ARE THE BENEFITS OF PHYSICAL ACTIVITY?

Individuals with disabilities are often less active than those without disabilities, yet they are at risk of the same health problems and also problems related to their disability, such as fatigue, obesity, lack of self-esteem, and social exclusion. There is a wealth of evidence to show that participation in physical activity for those with a disability can lead to improved levels of both physical health (such as cardiovascular fitness and strength) and psychological well-being (such as self-confidence, social awareness and self-esteem). In other words, physical activity can play an important role in the lives of those with disabilities, just as it can for those without disabilities. Before beginning any programme of physical activity, however, it is always a good idea to consult with the disabled individual to highlight any restrictions there may be.

INTERACTION

For those who are supervising activities it is often not the ability to adapt the activity that is the problem. In fact, problems normally arise when interacting with individuals with disabilities. Even though the list of disabilities is endless, there are certain ones that supervisors might come across that can be grouped together for the purpose of simplicity. These areas include: wheelchair use; hearing, speech or vision impairment and learning disability. The use of simple guidelines related to each of these areas can be helpful.

WHEELCHAIR USERS

One of the main misconceptions surrounding wheelchair use is that only those with mobility problems use wheelchairs. Just pop to your local sports centre and you will see non-disabled people using wheelchairs in a variety of sports. In statistical terms, fewer than 8% of disabled people

Wheelchair users: Interaction guidelines

- Any equipment a person may use, such as a wheelchair, is part of that person's personal space.
- Don't physically interact with an individual's body or equipment unless you're asked to do so or you ask first.
- When speaking with someone in a wheelchair, try to be at their eye level without kneeling.
- If a person transfers out of a wheelchair, to a car for example, leave the wheelchair within easy reach.
- Remind people to drink regularly as overheating often occurs.
- Encourage changing seat position often as circulation may be poor.

are wheelchair users. The use of wheelchairs in sporting situations can be traced back to the late 1940s when a German neurologist, the late Sir Ludwig Guttmann, introduced sport as part of the rehabilitation of his patients at the National Spinal Injuries Centre at Stoke Mandeville Hospital. In 1948 he organised the first national competition, which eventually led to the first Summer Paralympic Games (translated as games running in parallel) in 1960, in Rome. Guttmann is now widely acknowledged as the father of the Paralympic Games and sport for the disabled.

SPEECH IMPAIRMENT

Contrary to common belief, speech disabilities are hardly ever related to intelligence, so it is important not to treat them as such. Take the case of a person who has had a stroke, for example. In this case the effect can lead to the individual being severely hard of hearing or having a speech disability that others may find difficult to understand.

Speech impairment: Interaction guidelines

- Be patient when communicating.
- Don't speak for the person. Allow them to answer in their own time.
- Sometimes short questions (or 'closed questions' – those requiring a yes or no answer – as they are known) that require short answers or a nod or shake of the head are recommended.
- Never pretend to understand if you do not. Just be honest.

Hearing impairment: Interaction guidelines

- To get their attention, tap the person on the shoulder or wave your hand in front of them.
- Find out if the person prefers sign language, gesturing, writing or speaking.
- Look directly at the person, and speak clearly and slowly.
- Speak in a normal tone of voice.
- Try to talk when background noise is low.
- Face the sun if you are outside and try to have light on your face if you are inside.
- Written notes can often help. Do not talk while writing.
- If you have trouble understanding, just let the person know.

HEARING IMPAIRMENT

The range of hearing impairment is vast. This is easily evidenced as this particular disability can range from mild hearing loss to what is considered to be 'profound deafness' (which just means totally deaf). Some individuals who have only a mild degree of hearing loss might rely on the use of hearing aids, whereas others might rely on speech reading (lip reading), sign language, or a combination of both. According to the English Federation of Disability Sport, there are approximately 9 million deaf and hard of hearing people in the UK.

VISION IMPAIRMENT

As with hearing impairment, there is a wide range of vision impairment. Some individuals may only have limited vision and just require the use of

> **Vision impairment: Interaction guidelines**
> - Always identify yourself and others when meeting someone with vision impairment.
> - It helps to tell the person that the conversation has finished and you are moving.
> - When you give help, allow the person to take your arm so you can lead.
> - When offering a seat, place the person's hand on the back or arm of the seat.
> - Try to be consistent in each session with things like leaving equipment in the same place.
> - Use 'clock clues' to aid orientation in the room.
> - Use large print when writing or giving notes.

> **Learning disability: Interaction guidelines**
> - Be patient and make sure you understand.
> - Use precise and simple language.
> - Try to use words that relate to things around you that you both can see.
> - Try to give the same information in different ways.
> - If you are not sure about the response, repeat the question in a different way.
> - Give exact step-by-step instructions.
> - Ask the person if they prefer information in a verbal or written format.
> - Give constant reminders, such as to drink water and use sun cream regularly.

corrective lenses (glasses or contact lenses), whereas other individuals may have a total loss of vision. In the case of total loss of vision, the amount of dependence on others to help with daily activities can vary dramatically between individuals, from the use of a cane or stick to guide dogs or carer assistance.

LEARNING DISABILITY

A learning disability is a condition in which the brain does not develop as it should, and may occur as a result of brain injuries, infections, trauma, genetic or developmental problems, or difficulties with speech and language. Unfortunately there is often a 'stigma' attached to the term 'learning difficulties' but this is an extremely common condition as it is estimated that there are approximately 1.5 million people in the UK who have a learning disability, and about 200 babies are born with a learning disability every year. It is also an area that is rapidly gaining more awareness, which it is to be hoped will help reduce the negative connotations. According to the English Federation of Disability Sport, about 17% of people with a learning disability are employed, but more disturbing is the statistic that about nine out of ten people with a learning disability are bullied.

BENEFITS OF PHYSICAL ACTIVITY

The benefits of physical activity for those with disabilities can be physiological or psychological, and can be associated with either physical or mental health disabilities. In terms of those people with physical disabilities, the benefits of physical activity are almost identical to those for non-disabled people, taking into account the specific impact of the disability. In terms of mental health problems, according to the English Federation of Disability Sport they are now the UK's highest cause of time off work, with nearly three out of ten employees suffering a stress or mental health-related problem every year. This is quite an important statistic considering that about 21% of people with a mental health condition are in employment and that the WHO estimates that, by 2020, depression will become the second most important cause of disability in the world. Even though the effects of physical activity on mental health conditions are not fully understood, it is generally thought that there will be a beneficial effect in most cases. This supports the view of the ACSM that depression often accompanies a disability but can be improved by physical activity.

ACTIVITY GUIDELINES

Many individuals with disabilities regularly take part in organised sports or activities. As with anyone, cardiovascular capacity and muscular strength and endurance are components of fitness that should be addressed to help with the particular chosen sport or activity. For example, there are wheelchair variations that are now available for sports such as cycling, distance events, basketball, tennis and even skiing. It is obvious that these are all activities that require specific components of fitness to be developed. In terms of developing cardiovascular capacity, there are now many health or fitness centres that have machines that are adaptable for this specific purpose. For muscular strength and endurance training the use of free weights, resistance bands and resistance machines (these can provide support while lifting) are all effective. Although there are many different cardiovascular and resistance exercises that can be done, depending on the equipment available, there are some typical exercises for wheelchair users that can be done with equipment commonly found in most fitness centres. Figs 16.1 to 16.3 give a description of some of the cardiovascular exercises that can be done.

ARM CRANKING

There are many types of arm-cranking cardio machines in gyms nowadays. The user sits in the seat of the machine and uses their arms to turn the crank (a bit like pedals on a bike).

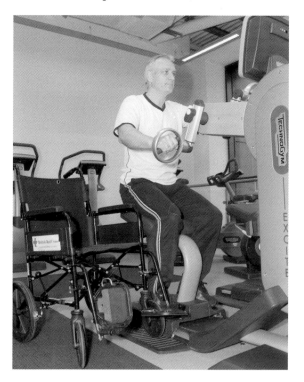

Figure 16.1 Arm cranking

ROWING/KAYAKING

Some rowing machines can now be adapted to fix the seat in place so that rowing can take place. There are also machines that are kayaking specific.

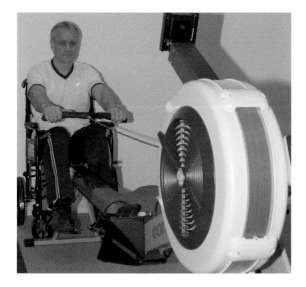

Figure 16.2 Rowing

DISTANCE 'WHEELING'

Wheelchairs with three wheels are now available to enable the user to do any type of distance event. These wheelchairs make it possible for the person to steer while maintaining speed.

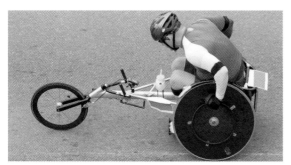

Figure 16.3 Wheeling

The range of resistance-type exercises that wheelchair users can do with resistance bands or free weights is endless. With resistance machines, however, this will depend on availability at the centre of choice. Figures 16.4 to 16.8 give a description of the more common resistance exercises that can be done with certain resistance machines, or in this particular case resistance bands if machines are not available.

Lat pull-down

1   To work the large muscles of the back, sit at a lat pull-down machine and extend the arms to take hold of the bar or a resistance band wrapped around any fixed point.
2   Pull the bar or bands down to chin level.
3   Extend the arms to the start position, controlling the movement all the way.

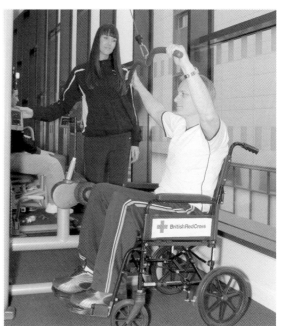

Figure 16.4 Lat pull-down

Chest press

1 To work the large muscles of the chest, sit at a bench or chest press machine and take hold of the handles or resistance band.
2 Extend the arms forwards until they are at full extension.
3 Let the arms return to the start point, but control the movement all the way.
4 At the start point try to keep the hands within peripheral vision as this will protect the shoulder joint.

Shoulder press

1 To work the muscles of the shoulder sit at a shoulder press machine and take hold of the handles or the resistance band that is passed under the seat.
2 Extend the arms above the head.
3 Let the arms return to the start point, but control the movement all the way.
4 For the start point, try to keep the upper arms parallel with the floor.

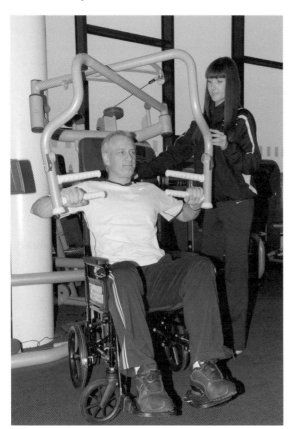

Figure 16.5 Chest press

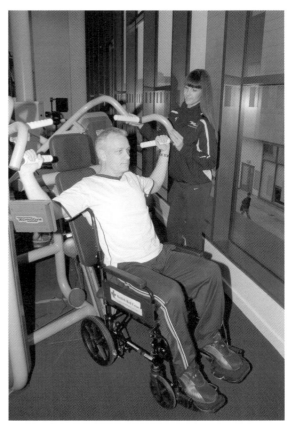

Figure 16.6 Shoulder press

Triceps push

1   To work the muscles at the back of the arms, sit at a triceps push machine and push down on the handles or the resistance band that is anchored overhead.
2   Control the arm movement back to the start position.

Biceps curl

1   To work the muscles of the front of the arms, sit at a biceps curl machine, take hold of the handles or bands and lift them towards the face.
2   Control the arm movement back to the start position.

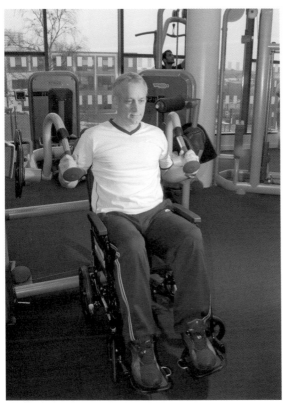

Figure 16.7 Triceps push

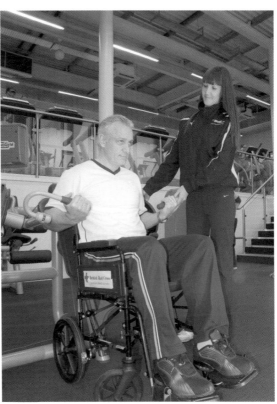

Figure 16.8 Biceps curl

For those that are not familiar with resistance training, especially with the use of resistance machines, there are a few general guidelines that can be followed.

- Take advice from a qualified instructor when selecting the appropriate weight for each exercise.
- Some makes of machine allow for the seat to be removed so that the wheelchair can be used as the seat.
- If the wheelchair is to be used, make sure that the individual is correctly strapped in.
- For resistance band exercises, make sure that the band is taut at the starting point of each exercise. Bands come in different thicknesses.

- Grip is often a problem for those with certain disabilities. The use of straps or 'action gloves' can be helpful.
- Try to identify muscles that are weak. These usually include latissimus dorsi, erector spinae and trapezius.

WHAT TESTS ARE THERE?

For many disabilities there are no specifically designed tests as most standard fitness tests are suitable depending on the particular disability. However, because of the lower body limitations that are often associated with wheelchair users, aerobic capacity is a component of fitness that is

---

Test box: Wheelchair fitness test

Equipment needed
Stopwatch, cones, track or measured distance.

1   Place cones around a track at 50 m intervals to aid measuring.
2   All participants line up on the start line.
3   Participants have to wheel around the track as far as they can for 12 minutes.
4   Record the distance to the nearest 100 m.

Use table 16.3 to give a fitness rating and an estimate of VO_2.

Table 16.3	Wheelchair fitness classifications		
Miles	**Kilometres**	**Estimated VO_2 (ml/kg/min)**	**Fitness rating**
<0.63	<1.01	<7.7	Poor
0.63–0.86	1.01–1.38	7.7–14.5	Below average
0.87–1.35	1.39–2.17	14.6–29.1	Fair
1.36–1.59	2.18–2.56	29.2–36.2	Good
>1.59	>2.56	>36.2	Excellent

commonly tested. There are various methods that have been used over the years, but one such test designed by Franklin *et al.* (1990), known as the 'wheelchair fitness test' (see previous page), allows the individual to be tested in their own wheelchair. The test does allow for an estimation of fitness rating and classification, however it is also useful for setting a baseline for the individual that can be used to track any future improvement.

RECOMMENDED READING

Active Living Alliance for Canadians with a Disability (1995) *Moving to inclusion*. Oxon Hill, MD: AAHPERD Publications (800-321-0789)

BAALPE (1996) *Physical education for children with special educational needs in mainstream education*. Leeds: White Line Press

De Pauw, K.P. & Gavron, S.J. (2005) *Disability and sport*. Champaign, IL: Human Kinetics

Franklin, B.A., Swantek, K.I., Grais, S.L., Johnstone, K.S., Gordon, S. & Timmis, G.C. (1990) Field test estimation of maximal oxygen consumption in wheelchair users. *Archives of Physical Medical Rehabilitation*, 71: 574–578

Lammertse, D. (2001) Maintaining health long-term with spinal cord injuries. *Topics in Spinal Cord Injury Rehabilitation*, 6(3): 1–21

Lockette, K. & Keys, A. (1994) *Conditioning with physical disabilities*. Champaign, IL: Human Kinetics

Miller, P.D. (1995) *Fitness programming and physical disability*. Champaign, IL: Human Kinetics

Peterson, P.A. & Quarstein, V.A. (2001) Disability awareness training for disability professionals. *Disability Rehabilitation*, 23(1): 43–48

Potempa, K., Braun, L.T., Tinknell, T. & Popovich, J. (1996) Physiological outcomes of aerobic exercise training in hemi paretic stroke patients. *Stroke*, 21(4): 101–105

Randazzo, D. & Corless, K. (1998) *Activity for everyone: Children of all abilities in a regular physical activity program*. Oxon Hill, MD: AAHPERD Publications

Rimmer, J. & Hedman, G. (1998) A health promotion program for stroke survivors. *Topics in Stroke Rehabilitation*, 5(2): 30–44

Rimmer, J.H. (1994) *Fitness and rehabilitation programs for special populations*. Dubuque, IA: WCB Brown & Benchmark

Seaman, J.A. (1995) *Physical best and individuals with disabilities: A handbook for inclusion in fitness testing*. Reston, VA: AAHPERD Publications

Sherrill, C. (1998) *Adapted physical activity and sport* (5th edn). Boston, MA: WCB McGraw-Hill

Special Olympics International (1997) *Fact sheet: Milestones*. Washington, DC: Special Olympics International

Wells, C. & Hooker, S. (1990) The spinal injured athlete. *Adapted Physical Activity Quarterly*, 7(3): 265–285

Winnick, J.P. (2005) *Adapted physical education and sport*. Champaign, IL: Human Kinetics

World Health Organization (2000) *ICF: International classification of functioning, disability and health*. Geneva: WHO Press

USEFUL WEBSITES

Association for Physical Education – www.afpe.org.uk

British Blind Sport – www.afpe.org.uk

British Deaf Sports Council – www.britishdeafsportscouncil.org.uk

CP Sport England & Wales – www.cpsport.org

Disability Sport England – www.disabilitysport.org.uk

Disability Sport Wales – www.disabilitysportwales.org

Disability Sports NI (Northern Ireland) – www.dsni.co.uk

Down's Syndrome Association – www.downs-syndrome.org.uk

English Federation of Disability Sport – www.efds.co.uk

ParalympicsGB – www.paralympics.org.uk

Scottish Disability Sport – www.scottishdisabilitysport.com/sds

UK Sports Association for People with Learning Disability – www.uksportsassociation.org

WheelPower (British Wheelchair Sports Foundation) – www.wheelpower.org.uk

ANTE- AND POSTNATAL

17

KEYPOINTS

- Pregnancy can be split roughly into equal three-month time periods called the first, second and third trimesters.
- The symptoms of pregnancy are not always present and not always consistent.
- There are many changes that can occur in the body as a result of pregnancy, such as cardiovascular, respiratory, metabolic, hormonal and body temperature changes.
- The separation of the rectus abdominis muscle is known as 'diastasis recti' and occurs in about two-thirds of all pregnant women.
- There is currently a debate as to whether or not there is an increased release of a hormone called relaxin during pregnancy. The effect of this particular hormone is thought to be to loosen ligaments throughout the pregnancy and up to 6 months after the birth.
- Even though the evidence is limited, it has been shown that there are potential benefits of physical activity for pregnant women.
- There are many associated risks of physical activity when pregnant and shortly afterwards that need to be considered.
- There are guidelines available for physical activity before, during and after pregnancy, but those supervising should be mindful of the signs to indicate that physical activity should stop (contraindications).

WHAT IS IT?

Pregnant women represent a unique clientele with regard to the health and fitness environment. Pregnancy can be split roughly into equal three-month time periods called 'trimesters', as can be seen in fig 17.1. This is referred to as the 'ante-natal' period. When a woman has given birth, the period up to about a year afterwards is known as the 'postnatal' period.

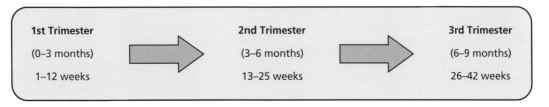

Figure 17.1 Approximate duration of trimesters

Table 17.1	Common symptoms associated with trimesters	
First trimester	**Second trimester**	**Third trimester**
• There is an increase in resting heart rate (5–10 bpm) and breathing rate, which in turn increases the metabolic rate • The woman undergoes hormonal changes such as the release of relaxin, which allows ligaments to stretch • The breasts and the uterus enlarge • Women gain on average about 1–3 kg	• Hormones tend to stabilise during this period • The intestinal tract relaxes • Colustrum secretion from the breasts • Linea nigra develops (dark vertical line on the abdomen) • The women can suffer bleeding gums • Backache due to postural changes • Weight gain on average is about 6–8 kg	• Women can become tired very easily • Some women develop high blood pressure • 'Braxton Hicks' contractions occur • Women can become anxious and not sleep well • Weight gain on average is about 3–4 kg • Venous return (blood flow back to the heart) can be reduced

There are many symptoms associated with pregnancy, most of which are uncomfortable but are generally a sign of a healthy pregnancy. Symptoms are not always present and are not always consistent, but generally speaking there are common symptoms that occur within each trimester, as shown in table 17.1.

ASSOCIATED CHANGES

There are many changes that take place early on within a pregnancy that cause the common symptoms. These changes, however, are essential for many different reasons such as making sure that a constant supply of energy to the foetus and mother is always available. The changes in the body can be grouped into several areas, such as cardiovascular, respiratory, metabolic, hormonal and body temperature changes. Table 17.2 gives a brief description of some of the changes that can occur.

Table 17.2	Typical changes associated with pregnancy
Changes	**Description**
Cardiovascular changes	
Blood volume increases	The volume of blood in the body can increase by as much as 30–40%, for obvious reasons
Red blood cell mass increases	Red blood cells can also increase by as much as 20–30% in order to supply oxygen to the foetus
Blood vessel walls dilate	The size of the blood vessels increases to allow greater blood flow, which results in something known as vascular underfill
Resting heart rate rises	RHR can rise by as much as 10–15 bpm
Cardiac output increases	The amount of blood pumped out of the heart every minute can increase by about 30%
The left ventricle enlarges	The chamber in the heart that pumps blood to the body can enlarge by about 20%
Blood flow to the skin increases	This occurs to help cool the body
Respiratory changes	
Increased ventilation rate and depth	This just means that breathing increases and the amount of air taken in and out (tidal volume) increases by about 40–50%
The brain is more sensitive to levels of carbon dioxide	This is partly responsible for the increase in breathing rate
Decreased residual volume	The amount of 'spare' space in the lungs decreases
Increased oxygen consumption	The amount of oxygen that is used up from the air increases by up to about 30%
Hyperventilation can occur	This can be common at about 12 weeks due to the release of the hormone progesterone
Metabolic adaptations	
Resting metabolic rate increases	The amount of energy used in the body at rest can increase by up to 20%
Symptoms of mild diabetes	This is due to a delayed insulin response
Carbohydrate energy supplies preferentially used by foetus	There is a high usage of carbohydrate by the foetus
Maternal blood sugar levels dip	This happens about every 6–8 hours due to usage by the foetus
Hormonal changes	
Relaxin release	This is released from ovaries up to about 12 weeks when it is released from the placenta; it can loosen ligaments postnatal for up to 6 months

Table 17.2	Typical changes associated with pregnancy (continued)
Changes	**Description**
Oestrogen release	
Progesterone release	The levels tend to remain high throughout pregnancy as it promotes foetal growth, causes breast enlargement and stimulates colostrum
	The levels are high throughout pregnancy as it relaxes smooth muscle, stabilises blood pressure and stimulates colostrum; greater insulin sensitivity to glucose can occur due to hormone level increase
Body temperature changes	
Mother's core temperature goes up	Temp can increase by 0.6°C at the start, and remain elevated for about 20 weeks
Pregnant glow	Some areas of skin become hotter by up to 2–6°C
Increase in heat loss	In early pregnancy heat dissipation is increased by up to 30% and in late pregnancy by up to 70% due to increased body mass
Quicker sweating	Because the blood flow to skin increases and the breathing rate elevates, both increasing heat loss

POSTURE CHANGES

As the baby gets bigger during pregnancy, it causes the centre of gravity of the mother to move. Generally speaking, the centre of gravity lies at the level of the naval just in front of the spine (except in those women who are pregnant). In the case of a pregnant woman, the baby is growing outwards, which causes the centre of gravity to move outwards and slightly down. As a result of this movement of the centre of gravity, there are several effects that can occur when pregnant; these can lead to back pain in many cases. Changes include the following:

* lengthening and weakening of abdominal muscles
* ligaments loosen, mainly around the hips, lower back and pelvis
* as a result of weakened muscles there is reduced support for the spine
* this weakness also causes an increased lumbar lordosis (hollow lower back) and an increased thoracic kyphosis (rounded upper back)
* the pelvis can also tilt forwards, which also increases the lumbar curve.

DIASTASIS RECTI

One of the main trunk muscles to be affected by pregnancy is the rectus abdominis, which runs from both sides of the lower ribs to the pelvic bone. During pregnancy this muscle lengthens and also becomes wider. When this occurs, the muscle might appear to split down the middle, as can be seen in fig 17.2, but it is actually a band of tendon (or aponeurosis) called the linea alba that separates

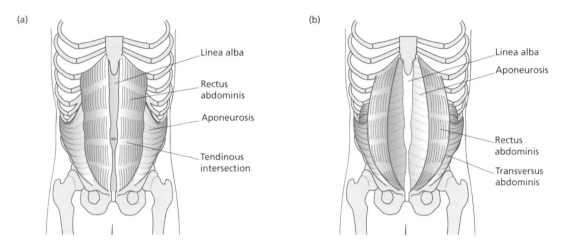

(a)

Linea alba

Rectus abdominis

Aponeurosis

Tendinous intersection

(b)

Linea alba

Aponeurosis

Rectus abdominis

Transversus abdominis

Figure 17.2 Abdominal wall before and after diastasis recti

to allow for growth of the baby. This separates to allow for growth of the baby. This separation of the rectus abdominis muscle is otherwise known as 'diastasis recti' and occurs in about two-thirds of all pregnant women.

During pregnancy there is also an increased release of a hormone called relaxin. The effect of this particular hormone is thought to be to loosen ligaments throughout the pregnancy and up to six months after the birth, although it is still a topic of debate whether this actually occurs or not. Because of the shift in centre of gravity and the effect of the relaxin, the loose ligaments supporting the pelvis, hips and lower back can stretch, leading to decreased stability and increased mechanical stress. It is important, therefore, that the muscles around the trunk and hips are kept as strong as possible and that any flexibility exercises at this point are stopped or done with extreme care.

PHYSICAL ACTIVITY BENEFITS

Much of the information in this chapter has been adapted from two main sources: the Royal College of Obstetricians and Gynaecologists (RCOG) and the American Congress of Obstetricians and Gynecologists (ACOG), which agree that physical activity during an uncomplicated pregnancy should be actively recommended for a host of maternal and foetal benefits. The amount of research relating to the area of ante- and postnatal physical activity is limited compared to other populations, as it is often difficult to carry out research on pregnant women. There is, however, a small amount of research that has been done as well as a huge amount of anecdotal evidence (word of mouth) as childbirth is obviously very common. The benefits of doing regular physical activity during pregnancy can be slightly different depending on the trimester – as can be seen in table 17.3, which outlines some of the potential benefits adapted from the RCOG and the ACOG.

As far as benefits to the foetus are concerned, research by Paisley *et al.* (2003) has suggested that the foetuses of exercising women tolerate labour better than the foetuses of non-exercising women. It has also been shown, such as in the investigation

Table 17.3 Potential benefits of physical activity for pregnant women

First trimester	Second trimester	Third trimester	Postnatal
• Reduce or alleviate symptoms of pregnancy	• Increased energy levels and reserves • Improved digestion • Reduced weight gain (fat) • Reduced back pain • Enhanced maternal well-being	• Increased self-esteem • Better posture • Improved sleep • More energy • Shorter and easier labour	• Leaner baby • Faster return to pre-pregnancy weight and fitness

Table 17.4 An Apgar score chart

Apgar sign	2	1	0
Heart rate	Normal (above 100 beats per minute)	Below 100 beats per minute	Absent (no pulse)
Breathing (rate and effort)	Normal rate and effort, good cry	Slow or irregular breathing, weak cry	Absent (no breathing)
Grimace (responsiveness)	Pulls away, sneezes, or coughs with stimulation	Facial movement only (grimace) with stimulation	Absent (no response to stimulation)
Activity (muscle tone)	Active, spontaneous movement	Arms and legs flexed with little movement	No movement, 'floppy' tone
Appearance (skin colour)	Normal colour all over (hands and feet are pink)	Normal colour (but hands and feet are bluish)	Bluish-grey or pale all over

by Clapp (2000), that foetal stress levels are lower in women who exercise throughout pregnancy (at 50% of their pre-conception level) compared to well-conditioned athletes who discontinued exercise before the end of their first trimester. Stress levels in the foetus were measured in several ways. One of the methods used is known as an Apgar test. This clinical test was developed by Virginia Apgar in 1952; it was designed to evaluate a newborn's physical condition just after birth and to determine any immediate need for extra medical or emergency care. The test is normally done twice: once at 1 minute after birth then again 5 minutes after birth. Table 17.4 is an adapted version of the Apgar test, which covers five main areas: activity and muscle tone, pulse (heart rate), grimace response (medically known as 'reflex irritability'), appearance (skin colouration) and respiration (breathing rate and effort). Each area is scored on a scale of 0 to 2 with 2 being the highest. When all areas are added together it gives a potential maximum score of 10 and potential minimum score of 0. A score of 7 or above after 1 minute is considered good. Anything less may just mean that the baby requires immediate attention. A score of less than 7 after 5 minutes usually means that the baby will require further medical care. It must be pointed out, however, that the test is not meant to predict long-term health as a low Apgar score is normal for some newborn babies.

PHYSICAL ACTIVITY RISK

Even though there are many benefits of a regular physical activity programme right through pregnancy and for the postnatal period (as there are with all populations), there are many associated risks that need to be considered. Again, even though the research information in this area is limited, a common-sense approach to err on the side of caution is highly recommended. Table 17.5 outlines some of the risks to pregnant women associated with physical activity, adapted from those published by the RCOG and the ACOG.

Anecdotally, there appears to be common concern that pregnancy will affect the mother psychologically as well as physiologically, although the concerns tend to change from ante- to postnatal stages. For example, some of the more common psychological effects in the early stages of pregnancy include overreacting to minor

Table 17.5	Potential risks of physical activity for pregnant women
Risk	**Explanation**
Increased risk of miscarriage	The risk of miscarriage is obviously higher as the amount and intensity of physical activity increases
Blood flow and oxygen delivery to the foetus is reduced	Oxygen is required to supply the working muscles doing the physical activity, which can be diverted away from the foetus
Hypotension	When lying on the back the foetus can press on blood vessels (the vena cava in particular) causing a loss of blood pressure
Umbilical cord problems	High-impact activities can result in the umbilical cord being wrapped around the foetus
Waters can break	High intensity or impact can cause waters to break
Extended or difficult labour	If abdominal and pelvic floor muscles are too strong they can in some cases extend the labour period
Poor breast milk	Strenuous exercise has been shown in some cases to reduce the quantity and quality of the mother's breast milk
Hyperthermia	The body temperature can rise more than it would normally, and excessive temperature (no more than 39.2°C) could affect the baby's development
Venous return reduction	In the third trimester, blood flow back to the heart can be reduced by the pressure on the inferior vena cava, especially in the supine position

situations and being prone to mood swings, as well as loss of self-esteem because of concern over bodily changes (such as an increase in weight and, in fewer cases, varicose veins). As the pregnancy goes on into the later stages there are often concerns over the ability to cope and feelings of being anxious about the delivery.

PHYSICAL ACTIVITY GUIDELINES

Any pregnant woman wishing to start a programme of regular physical activity should always obtain clearance from their doctor or physician prior to starting. Anyone wishing to supervise activity in the antenatal stage should make sure that they are qualified to do so by undertaking one of the many courses that are available. Once individuals are qualified to supervise physical activity for this population, they should become familiar with specific written questionnaires (known as screening forms) that are used to help identify pregnancies in which the risk of abnormality is higher than usual. One such screening form is the PARmed-X for PREGNANCY, which is available from the Canadian Society for Exercise Physiology. As far as general activity guidelines are concerned, it is suggested that if women are reasonably active prior to becoming pregnant, and are generally healthy, then there should be no problems in continuing recommended activity throughout the pregnancy. However, if the individual was sedentary prior to becoming pregnant it is recommended that only low-intensity activity should be undertaken. More specific guidelines have been published by the RCOG and the

ACOG, however an overview of the guidelines is presented below.

- Use the talk test or Borg rate of perceived exertion (RPE) scale to determine exercise intensity.
- Do not exercise to the point of exhaustion.
- Do not exercise in the supine (on the back) position and no motionless standing.
- Dress in light, comfortable clothing and keep well hydrated.
- Ingest carbohydrate (30–50 g) prior to exercise.
- Avoid abdominal exercises.
- Maintain training heart rate under 140 bpm.
- Avoid high-impact activities.

Both the RCOG and the ACOG recommend using the Borg RPE scale because the increased resting heart and increased stroke volumes associated with pregnant women make the use of heart rate monitoring quite difficult to do. The ACOG has also published information relating to certain circumstances for when pregnant women should not do or should stop doing any form of physical activity. These circumstances are more commonly known as 'contraindications' to exercise. Table 17.6 lists the contraindications for which physical activity should not be undertaken, and also explains related situations in which any activity that is in progress should be stopped.

Even though some of these terms may be unfamiliar, if the intention is to supervise a physical activity programme for someone who is pregnant, then before any activity is undertaken the individual should be asked if they have any of the contraindications. This shouldn't be a problem as someone who is pregnant should have a good understanding of the terms. It is important also

Table 17.6	Contraindications and reasons to stop activity for pregnant women
Contraindications	**Reasons to stop activity**
• Pregnancy-induced hypertension	• Vaginal bleeding
• Cardiac disease	• Leakage of fluid (amniotic)
• Type 1 or 2 diabetes	• Sudden calf pain or swelling in the ankles, hands or face
• Chronic bronchitis or lung disease	
• Pre-term rupture of membrane	• Headaches or visual disturbances
• Premature labour during the prior or current pregnancy	• Fainting or dizziness
	• Palpitations or chest pain
• Incompetent cervix	• Persistent or painful contractions (more than 6–8 per hour)
• Persistent second or third trimester bleeding	
• Intra-uterine growth retardation	• Muscle weakness
• Anaemia and blood disorders	• Excessive shortness of breath
• Thyroid disease	• Insufficient weight gain (less than 1 kg per month) during last two trimesters
• Cardiac dysrhythmia (irregular heartbeat)	
• Placenta previa (covers the cervix)	• Excessive fatigue
• Heavy smoker (more than 20 per day)	• Abdominal or pelvic pain
• Morbid obesity or very underweight	• Reduced foetal movement
• Sedentary	
• Multiple pregnancies	

that the supervisor (or the individual) should constantly monitor the situation during all physical activity for circumstances that require the activity to be stopped immediately (as in table 17.6, as suggested by the ACOG) and in some cases to seek medical advice. According to the RCOG there are age-related heart rate training zones for aerobic-type activities that should be followed as a general guideline for women who have a history of being active. Table 17.7 is adapted from these guidelines.

As far as general guidelines for antenatal physical activity are concerned, table 17.8 provides an overview taken from a variety of sources such as the RCOG, the ACOG and the American College of Sports Medicine (ACSM). Note that activity should be progressed only between the 13th and 28th weeks.

Table 17.7	Aerobic heart rate training zones
Maternal age	**Heart rate target zone (beats/min)**
Less than 20 years	140–155
20–29 years	135–150
30–39 years	130–145
Over 40 years	125–140

Table 17.8	Physical activity guidelines for antenatal women	
	Aerobic training	**Strength training**
Mode	• Walking, cycling and water-based activities are good for this condition	• Continue as normal if already active; if not, slow progression from body weight to machines/free weights
Intensity	• RPE level 10–14 • 60–80%HRmax	• Avoid heavy loads • Overload by increasing repetitions
Duration	• 5–45 minutes per session • Increase by 2 mins per week but only between the 13th and 28th weeks	• Perform 1 to 3 sets of 15–20 RM • 1–2 minutes' rest between exercises
Frequency	Active person: • 3–4 per week up to 14th week • 3–5 per week up to 28th week • 3 per week after 28th week Non-active person: • None before 13th week • 3 per week 13th–36th weeks • 1–2 per week after 36th week	• 2–3 sessions per week • Encourage other forms of exercise • Decrease weight and sets, and increase recovery time as pregnancy progresses
Precautions	• Avoid high-impact activities and excessive repetition • Watch for signs of overheating	• If no experience prior to pregnancy, do not start • Avoid overstretching and overhead lifts

General precautions
- Non-active women are advised to seek medical approval before beginning a programme of activity.
- If any activity causes pain or discomfort, it should be stopped immediately.
- Do a rectus abdominis check 6–12 weeks after delivery (see opposite) before doing certain abdominal exercises.
- Be aware of episiotomy (see opposite) and take appropriate steps.
- Avoid motionless standing.
- Avoid supine exercises (lying on the back) after 16 weeks.

POSTNATAL ACTIVITY

It is essential that strengthening around the core (trunk) area is carried out throughout the pregnancy and afterwards, as the strain on this area due to the increased load of the baby is immense. Abdominal and back-strengthening exercises should be incorporated into all resistance training sessions. The pelvic floor muscle becomes particularly weak during pregnancy so needs particular attention, as it is responsible for bladder, uterus and rectum control. The pelvic floor muscle needs to be strengthened using exercises known as 'Kegal' exercises. The reason for this is that the pelvic floor muscle is stretched throughout pregnancy and delivery with the weight of the baby. These exercises can be done by squeezing the muscles that you use to stop the flow of urine. Hold for up to 10 seconds, then release. Do the exercises 10–20 times in a row at least three times a day.

One concern that must be taken into account before any exercise is done, however, is when an 'episiotomy' has been carried out. An episiotomy is the name given to a surgical procedure where an incision is made between the anus and the vagina to widen the exit route for the baby. If this has been done, then it usually takes about 10–15 days to heal and about 6 weeks for the stitches to dissolve. The other concern before doing any physical activity is related to the separation of the rectus abdominis muscle (or, more accurately, the linea alba). It is common that the rectus abdominis can separate by as much as 20 cm (a two- to three-finger gap) following delivery of the baby. It is important therefore that time is given to allow the muscle to return to its normal position. This usually takes a few weeks, so it is important not to do certain exercises, such as abdominal or oblique curls and sit-ups, in this time period. It is relatively easy for mothers to check their own rectus abdominis to see if it is realigned and that the linea alba has healed. This can be done by taking the following steps.

1   Lie on your back with knees bent and feet flat on the floor.
2   Slide a hand under the lower back to check the lumbar curve. The hand should fit snugly.
3   Raise the head and shoulders slightly off the floor (get someone to help if necessary) as this will cause the rectus abdominis to contract.
4   Run the fingers across the abdomen above and below the belly button, as in fig 17.3 opposite (with light pressure only).
5   Make sure you keep breathing throughout.

If the gap in the rectus abdominis is less than 3 cm (about two fingers wide), this is an indication that the linea alba has fully healed and that the rectus has realigned. If the gap is wider than this, it is recommended that certain abdominal exercises, such as abdominal or oblique curls and sit-ups, are *not* done as this could cause abdominal doming (which is a bulge in the abdominal wall). This is also the case with a Caesarean section, which is a surgical procedure that opens the abdomen and lower segment of the uterus to deliver a baby that cannot be born through the vagina. It is important to understand that if a mother has had a Caesarean section birth, abdominal exercises should not be done until the rectus abdominis has realigned and the wound is fully healed. This can take as long as 12 weeks to heal and, even then, exercises should be done carefully and with slow progression.

RECOMMENDED READING

American College of Obstetricians & Gynecologists (1994) ACOG Technical Bulletin No. 189: Exercise during pregnancy and the post-partum period. *International Journal of Gynecology and Obstetrics*, 45: 65–70

American College of Obstetricians & Gynecologists (2002) ACOG Committee Opinion No. 267: Exercise during pregnancy and the postpartum period. *Obstetrics and Gynecology*, 99: 171–173

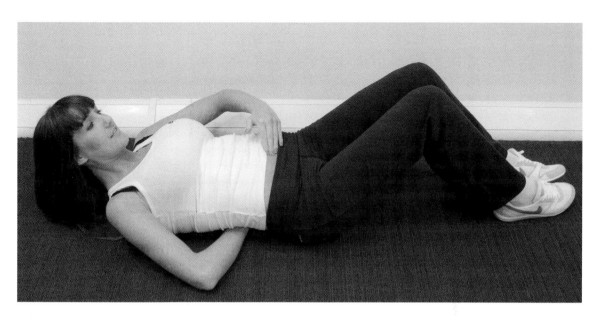

Figure 17.3 Checking the rectus abdominis

American College of Sports Medicine (2009) *ACSM's guidelines for exercise testing and prescription* (8th edn). London: Lippincott Williams & Wilkins

American Congress of Obstetricians & Gynecologists (2003a) *Exercise during pregnancy. ACOG patient education.* Washington, DC: ACOG

American Congress of Obstetricians & Gynecologists (2003b) *Getting in shape after your baby is born. ACOG patient education.* Washington, DC: ACOG

Artal, R. & O'Toole, O. (2003) Guidelines of the American College of Obstetricians and Gynecologists for exercise during pregnancy and the postpartum period. *British Journal of Sports Medicine*, 37: 6–12

Avery, N.D., Stocking, K.D., Tranmer, J.E., Davies, G.A. & Wolfe, L.A. (1999) Fetal responses to maternal strength and conditioning exercises in late gestation. *Canadian Journal of Applied Physiology*, 24: 362–376

Bauer, P.W., Broman, C.L. & Pivarnik, J.M. (2004) Exercise and pregnancy survey for health care providers. *Medicine and Science in Sports and Exercise*, 36(5): Abstract S113

Clapp, J.F. (2000) Exercise during pregnancy. A clinical update. *Clinical Sports Medicine*, 19: 273–286

Clapp, J.F., Kim, H., Burcio, B., Schmidt, S., Petry, K. & Lopez, B. (2002) Continuing regular exercise during pregnancy: Effect of exercise volume on fetoplacental growth. *American Journal of Obstetrics and Gynecology*, 186: 142–147

Clarke, P.E. & Gross, H. (2004) Women's behaviour, beliefs and information sources about physical exercise in pregnancy. *Midwifery*, 20: 133–141

Da Costa, D., Rippen, N., Dritsa, M. & Ring, A. (2003) Self-reported leisure-time physical activity during pregnancy and relationship to psychological well-being. *Journal of Psychosomatic Obstetrics and Gynaecology*, 24: 111–119

Davies, G.A., Wolfe, L.A., Mottola, M.F. & MacKinnon, C. (2003) Joint SOGC/CSEP clinical practice guideline: Exercise in pregnancy and the postpartum period. *Journal of Obstetrics and Gynaecology Canada*, 25: 516–529

Dempsey, J.C., Butler, C.L. & Williams, M.A. (2005) No need for a pregnant pause: Physical activity may reduce the occurrence of gestational diabetes mellitus and preeclampsia. *Exercise and Sport Sciences Reviews*, 33(3): 141–149

Dempsey, J.C., Sorensen, T.K., Williams, M.A., Lee, I.M., Miller, R.S., Dashow, E.E. & Luthy, D.A. (2004)

Prospective study of gestational diabetes mellitus risk in relation to maternal recreational physical activity before and during pregnancy. *American Journal of Epidemiology*, 159: 663–670

Evenson, K.R., Savitz, D.A. & Huston, S.L. (2004) Leisure-time physical activity among pregnant women in the US. *Paediatric and Perinatal Epidemiology*, 118: 4000–4007

Goodwin, A., Astbury, J. & McMeeken, J. (2000) Body image and psychological well-being in pregnancy. A comparison of exercisers and non-exercisers. *Australian and New Zealand Journal of Obstetrics and Gynaecology*, 40: 422–447

Kardel, K.R. & Kase, T. (1998) Training in pregnant women: Effects on fetal development and birth. *American Journal of Obstetrics and Gynecology*, 178: 280–286

Krans, E.E., Gearhart, J.G., Dubbert, P.M., Klar, P.M., Miller, A.L. & Replogle, W.H. (2005) Pregnant women's beliefs and influences regarding exercise during pregnancy. *Journal of the Mississippi State Medical Association*, 46(3): 67–73

Leiferman, J.A. & Evenson, K.R. (2003) The effect of regular leisure physical activity on birth outcomes. *Maternal and Child Health Journal*, 7: 59–64

Lokey, E.A., Tran, Z.V., Wells, C.L., Myers, B.C. & Tran, A.C. (1991) Effects of physical exercise on pregnancy outcomes: A meta-analytic review. *Medicine and Science in Sports and Exercise*, 23: 1234–1239

Lynch, A.M., McDonald, S., Magann, E.F., Evans, S.F., Choy, P.L., Dawson, B., Blanksby, B.A. & Newnham, J.P. (2003) Effectiveness and safety of a structured swimming program in previously sedentary women during pregnancy. *Journal of Maternal-Fetal and Neonatal Medicine*, 114(3): 163–169

MacPhail, A., Davies, G.A., Victory, R. & Wolfe, L.A. (2000) Maximal exercise testing in late gestation: Fetal responses. *Obstetrics and Gynecology*, 96: 565–570

Morris, S.N. & Johnson, N.R. (2005) Exercise during pregnancy: A critical appraisal of the literature. *Journal of Reproductive Medicine*, 50(3): 181–188

Paisley, T.S., Joy, E.A. & Price, R.J. (2003) Exercise during pregnancy: A practical approach. *Current Sports Medicine Reports*, 2: 325–330

Petersen, A.M., Leet, T.L. & Brownson, R.C. (2005) Correlates of physical activity among pregnant women in the United States. *Medicine and Science in Sports and Exercise*, 37: 1748–1753

Pivarnik, J.M., Chambliss, H.O., Clapp, J.F., Dugan, S.A., Hatch, M.C., Lovelady, C.A., Mottola, M.F. & Williams, M.A. (2006) Impact of physical activity during pregnancy and postpartum on chronic disease risk. *Medicine and Science in Sports and Exercise*, 38: 989–1006

Poudevigne, M.S. & O'Connor, P.J. (2006) A review of physical activity patterns in pregnant women and their relationship to psychological health. *Sports Medicine*, 36: 19–38

Sorensen, T.K., Williams, M.A., Lee, I.M., Dashow, E.E., Thompson, M.L. & Luthy, D.A. (2003) Recreational physical activity during pregnancy and risk of preeclampsia. *Hypertension*, 41: 1273–1280

Stevenson, L. (1997) Exercise in pregnancy. Part 2: Recommendations for individuals. *Canadian Family Physician*, 43: 107–111

Yeo, S., Steele, N.M., Chang, M.C., Leclaire, S.M., Ronis, D.L. & Hayashi, R. (2000) Effect of exercise on blood pressure in pregnant women with a high risk of gestational hypertensive disorders. *Journal of Reproductive Medicine*, 45(4): 293–298

Zeanah, M. & Schlosser, S.P. (1993) Adherence to ACOG guidelines on exercise during pregnancy: Effect on pregnancy outcome. *Journal of Obstetric, Gynecologic, and Neonatal Nursing*, 22: 329–335

USEFUL WEBSITES

American Congress of Obstetricians and Gynecologists – www.acog.org

Canadian Society for Exercise Physiology – www.csep.ca

Royal College of Obstetricians and Gynaecologists – www.rcog.org.uk

ASSOCIATED MEDICATION

18

This particular section is not a definitive guide to the prescribed medication related to the conditions covered within this book. This is because the research and development related to the associated medication is in a constant state of progression, and therefore any published information can become out of date very quickly. This section does, however, attempt to provide the reader with an understanding of the potential side effects related to specific medications, which might be useful when considering physical activity programmes.

Those supervising activities for a person who is taking prescribed medication for a particular condition should always consult a GP or specialist if they are in any way unsure. There are also online sources of information related to prescription drugs, such as the Mims website (www.mims.co.uk), the RxList internet drug index (www.rxlist.com) and the NHS website (www.nhs.uk). Tables 18.1 to 18.11 give an overview of the potential side effects of prescribed medication related to certain conditions.

Table 18.1	Typical medication for diabetes
Medication	**Effect**
Angiotensin-converting enzyme (ACE) inhibitor	Often recommended as the first choice for those with high blood pressure and those with signs of kidney disease; delays absorption of carbohydrate
Insulins	Mainly given to type I diabetics; can be given in synthetic form known as insulin analogues
Aspirin	To prevent heart disease in people with diabetes who: • are older than 40; • have a personal or family history of heart problems; • have high blood pressure or high cholesterol and • smoke.
Biguanides	Decreases the production of glucose
Glucosidase inhibitors	Prevents the absorption of glucose from the gut

Caution
ACE inhibitors can reduce blood pressure (watch out for hypotension), and cause bloating and diarrhoea.
Aspirin – can increase systolic blood pressure during exercise.

Table 18.2	Typical medication for chronic obstructive pulmonary disease(COPD)
Medication	**Effect**
Bronchodilators	Both short- and long-term bronchodilators (open the airways by relaxing the smooth muscle) via inhaled delivery as a preference
Corticosteroids	These are anti-inflammatory drugs which prevent the release of certain hormones, even though there is debate about the effectiveness with this condition

Caution
Corticosteroids have many side effects (see table 18.9).
Some bronchodilators can elevate heart rate and blood pressure.

Table 18.3	Typical medication for asthma
Medication	**Effect**
Short-acting beta$_2$-adrenoceptor agonists	These are classed as bronchodilators (open the airways by relaxing the smooth muscle) via inhaled, oral or injected delivery
Long-term control such as corticosteroids and leukotriene blockers	These are anti-inflammatory drugs, which prevent the release of certain hormones
Long-acting beta$_2$-agonists (LABD)	Similar to short acting but have a 12-hour effect

Caution
Some beta$_2$-adrenoceptor agonists can elevate heart rate and blood pressure, and cause tremors, headaches and muscle cramps.
Corticosteroids are associated with a sore throat and mouth infections, and long-term use can lead to osteoporosis and weight gain.

Table 18.4	Typical medication for hypertension
Medication	**Effect**
ACE inhibitors	These drugs work by lowering the amount of a chemical produced in the bloodstream called angiotensin II, which constricts (narrows) blood vessels
Calcium-channel blockers	These drugs affect the way calcium is used in the blood vessels and the heart, which ultimately has a relaxing effect on the blood vessels
Diuretics ('water tablets')	Bendroflumethiazide is a commonly used diuretic to treat hypertension; diuretics increase the amount of salt and fluid passed out in the urine, which results in a reduction in blood pressure
Beta blockers	These work by reducing the heart rate, and reducing the force of contraction of the heart, which in turn can lower the blood pressure

Caution
Beta blockers can impair the ability of the body to regulate temperature and can increase blood triglyceride levels.
Diuretics can cause dehydration and increase total cholesterol levels.

Table 18.5 — Typical medication for hyperlipidaemia

Medication	Effect
Statins	These medications work by reducing the production of LDL-cholesterol within the body
Fibrates	Mainly lower triglycerides
Bile-acid binders	Reduce the level of LDL-cholesterol by preventing absorption

Caution
Statins and fibrates may cause muscle damage.
Bile-acid binders and fibrates may cause gastrointestinal problems.

Table 18.6 — Typical medication for arthritis

Medication	Effect
Analgesics and non-steroidal anti-inflammatory drugs (NSAIDs)	Analgesics relieve pain, NSAIDs are a large class of medications useful against pain and inflammation; a number of NSAIDs are available over the counter; more than a dozen are available only with a prescription
Disease-modifying anti-rheumatic drugs (DMARDs)	They relieve painful, swollen joints and slow joint damage, and several DMARDs may be used over the disease course; they take a few weeks or months to have an effect but are contentious
Corticosteroids	These are steroids given by mouth or injection; they are used to relieve inflammation and reduce swelling, redness, itching and allergic reactions

Caution
NSAIDs can cause stomach irritation and affect kidney function; also associated with gastrointestinal problems including ulcers, bleeding and perforation of the stomach.
DMARDs may increase risk of infection, hair loss, and kidney or liver damage.
Corticosteroids may cause indigestion, nervousness, restlessness, diabetes and osteoporosis.

Table 18.7 — Typical medication for osteoporosis

Medication	Effect
Parathyroid hormone and vitamin D	Appropriate doses have been found to increase bone mass
Bisphosphonates	Prevent bone loss mainly in the hip and spine
Calcitonin	A naturally occurring hormone used to prevent bone loss
Oestrogen	Mixed results relating to slowing the progression of osteoporosis

Caution
Bisphosphonates can cause abdominal or musculoskeletal pain, nausea or heartburn (uncommon).
Calcitonin can sometimes bring on an allergic reaction to the injection.
Oestrogen can increase a woman's risk of developing cancer.

Table 18.8	Typical medication for Parkinson's disease
Medication	**Effect**
Dopaminergics such as levodopa	Help to increase levels of dopamine in order to reduce symptoms
Dopamine agonists	Help to stimulate the production of dopamine
COMT inhibitor	This is used in conjunction with levodopa as it can prolong its action

Caution
Dopaminergics, dopamine agonists and COMT inhibitor can all cause vomiting, nausea and drowsiness.

Table 18.9	Typical medication for multiple sclerosis
Medication	**Effect**
Interferon beta	Given long term by injection to try to reduce the number of attacks
Glatiramer acetate	Given long term by injection to try to reduce the number of attacks
Corticosteroids	Normally given during symptomatic attacks to relieve symptoms

Caution
Corticosteroid side effects include heart failure, high blood pressure, high blood sugar levels, high or low levels of sodium in the blood, low level of potassium in the blood, personality changes (e.g. mood swings), stomach ulcer and swelling (oedema) caused by fluid retention.
Interferon can cause liver damage and infertility.
Glatiramer acetate can bring on a post-injection reaction of palpitations and tight chest.

Table 18.10	Typical medication for cardiovascular disease (CVD)
Medication	**Effect**
Angiotensin-converting enzyme (ACE) inhibitors	Stop the production of a chemical that makes blood vessels narrow and are used to help control high blood pressure and for damaged heart muscle; it may be prescribed after a heart attack to help the heart pump blood better
Beta blockers and calcium channel blockers	Used mainly for angina patients to reduce heart rate and blood pressure, and make the heart work less by blocking the hormone adrenalin
Anticoagulants such as warfarin	Help to prevent blood clots
Antiplatelets such as aspirin	Can decrease the clotting ability of the blood
Diuretics	There are many different types that are used to reduce high blood pressure, and levels of LDL-cholesterol and triglycerides
Nitrates	Used for both relief and prevention of angina by making more oxygen available to the heart muscle

Caution
ACE inhibitors, beta and calcium channel blockers can all reduce heart rate and blood pressure (watch out for hypotension) but can also cause nausea, headaches, dizziness.
Beta blockers can raise blood glucose in those with diabetes and can cause cold extremities as well as sleep disturbances.
Calcium channel blockers can cause dizziness, ankle swelling and constipation.
Warfarin may make bleeding worse.
Aspirin can cause indigestion, nausea and vomiting.
Diuretics can cause diabetes, gout, rashes and gastrointestinal upset.
Nitrates can cause headache, dizziness and nausea.

Table 18.11	Typical medication for stroke
Medication	**Effect**
Statin	Used as it helps to lower cholesterol and reduce risk of further problems
Antiplatelets such as aspirin or clopidogrel	Recommended for those who have suffered an ischemic stroke to help prevent clots
Anticoagulants such as warfarin	Help to prevent blood clots in patients who have atrial fibrillation
Hypertension medication (see table 18.4)	Used to lower blood pressure as this is a major risk factor for strokes

Caution
Statin can cause gastrointestinal upset.
Warfarin may make bleeding worse.
Aspirin can cause indigestion, nausea and vomiting.

GLOSSARY

Acetyl coenzyme A – Produced from the breakdown of pyruvic acid.

Acetylcholine (ACh) – Neurotransmitter substance released from several types of neuron.

Actin – Protein structure within a muscle cell.

Adaptation – Change due to repeated stimuli such as resistance training.

Adenosine triphosphate (ATP) – Main energy currency of the cell.

Adrenaline – A neurotransmitter that can stimulate the breakdown of fat and glycogen.

Aerobic – In the presence of oxygen.

Aerobic fitness – The ability to deliver oxygen to the working muscles and use it during exercise.

Agility – A rapid whole-body movement with change of velocity or direction in response to a stimulus.

Agonist – Refers to a muscle or muscle group responsible for the main action.

Air-displacement plethysmography – Direct method of assessing body composition.

Alveoli – Air sac in the lungs.

Anaerobic – In the absence of oxygen.

Anaerobic capacity – The total amount of energy that can be produced anaerobically during a bout of exercise.

Anaerobic fitness – The ability to perform maximal-intensity exercise.

Anaerobic power – The maximal rate at which energy can be produced.

Anaerobic threshold – The point at which the energy demand of the exercise being carried out can no longer be met by the aerobic system.

Android – Distribution of fat around the middle of the body.

Angina – Severe chest pains.

Anhydrous – Has no water in it.

Ankylosing spondylitis – Inflammation of joints in the spine or sacrum.

Antagonist – Refers to a muscle or muscle group responsible for opposing the main action.

Anthropometry – The science relating to the measurement of body mass and proportions of the human body.

Aorta – The main artery leading away from the left ventricle.

Arrhythmia – Deviation from normal heartbeat.

Asthma – Type of obstructive lung disease.

Atherosclerosis – Narrowing and hardening of the arteries.

Atrial fibrillation – Disorganised contraction of the atria resulting in ineffective pumping of blood to the ventricle.

Atrium – Chamber in the heart that receives blood from blood vessels.

Autonomic nervous system – Neurons that are not under conscious control.

Avascular – Lack of blood supply.

Axon – Branch of a motor neuron.

Bioelectrical impedance – Indirect method of assessing body composition.

Blood pressure – The force of the blood on the artery walls.

BMI – Body mass index (weight divided by height squared).

Bradycardia – Low resting heart rate.

Bronchitis – Inflammation of the airways.

Bronchoconstriction – Type of obstructive lung disease.

Calorie – The amount of energy needed to increase the temperature of 1 g of water by 1°C.

Capillary – The smallest type of blood vessel.

Cardiac output – The amount of blood pumped out of each ventricle per minute.

Cardiovascular – Relating to the heart and associated vessels.

Cardiovascular disease – Disease of the heart (and related vessels).

Cell – Basic structural and functional unit of life.

Centre of gravity – The point at which the body can be balanced.

Cholesterol – A fat-like steroid used to form cell membranes.

Claudication – Painful feeling in the legs.

Co-contraction – Tension developed in an agonist and antagonist muscle.

Concentric contraction – A muscular contraction against a resistance in which the muscle length shortens.

Contraction – Electrical stimulation of muscle to shorten.

Correlation – The relationship between two measurements or groups of measurements.

Dehydration – Water loss from a state of normal amounts of body water.

Delayed onset muscle soreness – Perception of post-exercise soreness.

Densitometry – Direct method of assessing body composition.

Developmental stretch – A stretch held long enough to induce physical structure development to increase flexibility.

Diaphragm – Muscle used for breathing.

Diaphysis – The shaft of a bone.

Diastolic – The time between the ventricle contractions when it is filling.

Diffusion – Movement of molecules from high to low concentration in order to reach a uniform concentration.

Distal – The segment of the body furthest from the centre of the body.

Dyslipidaemia – Abnormal amount of lipids in the blood.

Dyspnoea – Shortness of breath.

Eccentric contraction – A muscular contraction against a resistance in which the muscle lengthens.

EIA – Exercise-induced asthma.

EIB – Exercise-induced bronchoconstriction.

Elasticity – The ability to resist deformation and return to the original shape.

Electrocardiogram (ECG) – Device used to record the electrical activity of the heart.

Emphysema – Destruction of the surface of the alveoli.

Endocrine system – An integrated system of organs, glands and tissues that involve the release of extracellular signalling molecules known as hormones.

Energy – The capacity to do work.

Energy system – A term used to describe the source or pathway of producing ATP.

Enzymes – Proteins that can speed up chemical reactions.

Epiphysis – A region towards the end of a bone known as a 'growth plate'.

Erythrocyte – A red blood cell.

Expired air – Air that is breathed out.

Extension – Movement at a joint in which the joint angle increases.

Extrinsic injury – An injury caused as a result of an external force.

Extrinsic motivation – The task leads to a reward.

Fascia – Type of connective tissue.

Fast twitch – Type of muscle fibre associated with strength and speed.

Flexibility – The available range of motion around a specific joint.

Flexion – Movement at a joint in which the joint angle decreases.

Forced expiratory ratio – The ratio between FVC and FEV_1.

Forced expiratory volume in 1 second – The volume of air exhaled during the first second of forced expiration.

Forced vital capacity – The volume of air exhaled during a forced maximal exhalation following a forced maximal inhalation.

Gland – A group of cells that release hormones.

Goniometry – Measurement of joint angles.

Gout – Joint inflammation caused by uric acid crystal deposits.

Gravity – Force of attraction caused by the Earth.

Gynoid – Distribution of fat around the hips and thighs.

Haemoglobin – Part of a red blood cell that carries oxygen or carbon dioxide.

Heart rate – The number of heart beats per minute.

High-density lipoprotein – Cholesterol transporters often referred to as 'good cholesterol' by transporting cholesterol to the liver to be broken down and excreted.

Histamine – A chemical in the body that has the effect of widening the airways.

Homeostasis – When the systems of the body are working optimally and within limits.

Hormone – A chemical messenger in the body.

HRmax – Maximum heart rate.

Hyperglycaemia – High levels of blood glucose.

Hyperlipidaemia – High levels of fat in the blood.

Hyperplasia – An increase in the number of muscle fibres.

Hypertension – High blood pressure.

Hypertrophy – Enlargement of an organ such as muscle.

Hypocapnia – Very low pressure of carbon dioxide in the blood.

Hypoglycaemia – Low levels of blood glucose.

Hypotension – Low blood pressure.

Hypothermia – A body temperature of below 34 or 35°C.

Hypoxia – Reduced oxygen supply to tissues.

Inspired air – Air that is breathed in.

Insulin – A hormone secreted by the pancreas, which reduces blood sugar levels.

Intensity – A measurement of the difficulty level, or 'hardness', of the exercise.

Internal rotation – Rotation of a part of the body towards the mid-point.

Intervertebral disc – Spongy collagenous disc between vertebrae that acts as a shock absorber.

Intrinsic injury – An injury caused as a result of internal forces.

Intrinsic motivation – The task itself brings about the reward.

Ischemia – A low oxygen state (normally due to blocked arteries).

Isometric contraction – Muscle contraction where there is no change in the muscle length.

Isotonic contraction – Muscle contraction against a constant load, as in free-weight training.

Ketones – Chemicals in the body regarded as toxins.

Kyphosis – Curvature of the thoracic spine.

Lactic acid – A waste product as a result of glycogen breakdown without the presence of oxygen.

Ligament – Tissue in the body that connects bone to bone, used for support.

Lipid – The overall term used to describe any fat-soluble molecule.

Lipolysis – Breakdown of triglyceride to fatty acids and glycerol.

Lordosis – Excessive primary curve of the lumbar spine.

Low-density lipoprotein – Known as 'bad cholesterol'. Tends to deposit cholesterol on blood vessel walls.

Lumen – The channel within a vessel or tube.

Lupus – An autoimmune disease that affects joints.

Mass – The quantity of matter a body contains.

Mast cell – Place in the body from which histamines are released.

Maximum heart rate (MHR) – Theoretically the maximum possible heart rate for an individual.

Metabolic equivalent (MET) – A method of expressing energy expenditure.

Metabolic rate – The amount of energy expended at a given time.

Metabolic syndrome – A combination of abdominal obesity, hypertension, dyslipidaemia and impaired fasting glucose.

Millimetres – A small unit of distance.

Mitochondria – The 'power cell' or site of aerobic energy production.

mmol – A minute amount. Often used when testing blood, etc.

Molecule – Two or more atoms joined together.

Motoneuron – Nerves that transmit signals away from the central nervous system to the muscles.

Multiple sclerosis – A chronic disease that affects nerve fibres.

Muscle spindle – Structures within muscle that detect changes in length.

Muscular endurance – The ability of a muscle or muscle group to perform repeated contractions against a resistance over a period of time.

Muscular strength – The maximum amount of force a muscle or muscle group can generate.

Myocardial infarction – Irreversible injury to the heart muscle.

Myocardium – Essentially the heart muscle.

Myofibril – The smallest muscle fibre.

Myosin – Protein structure within a muscle cell.

Neural – Relating to the nervous system.

Neuromuscular – Relating to the muscular and associated nervous system.

Noradrenaline – A stress hormone.

Obesity – The percentage body fat at which the risk to the individual of disease is increased.

Origin – The attachment point of a muscle to a bone nearest to the midline of the body.

Ossification – The process of bone growth.

Osteoarthritis – Inflammation due to erosion of bone surfaces.

Osteoblast – A bone-building cell.

Osteoclast – A bone-modelling cell.

Osteoporosis – A condition of reduced bone density.

Palpation – The part of a physical examination in which an object or subject is felt.

Pancreas – Organ in the body that secretes insulin.

Parasympathetic nervous system – Division of the autonomic nervous system that can slow the heart rate.

Parkinson's disease – A chronic disease related to movement disorder.

PAR-Q – The Physical Activity Readiness Questionnaire.

PEFR – Peak expiratory flow rate.

Perceived exertion – A subjective measurement of exercise intensity.

Periosteum – The tough outer layer of a long bone.

Peripheral vascular disease – Narrowing of arteries not related to the heart or brain.

Phosphate-creatine (PCr) – A chemical compound stored in the muscles.

Plasma – Major fluid component of blood in which blood cells are suspended.

Platelets – Clotting cells.

Pleura – A double-layered membrane surrounding the lungs.

Plyometric – Rapid eccentric loading followed by a brief isometric phase and explosive rebound using stored elastic energy and powerful concentric contractions.

POMS (Profile of Mood States) – Psychological questionnaire used to determine mood states.

Power – The product of force and velocity. Power = Work (force x distance) ÷ Time.

Prone – Lying on the front.

Proprioception – Sense of position in space.

Proprioceptive neuromuscular facilitation – A type of partner-assisted stretching.

Proximal – The segment of the body closest to the centre of the body.

Reciprocal inhibition – The term used to describe the amount of relaxation elicited in the antagonist muscle when the agonist muscle contracts.

Residual volume – The volume of gas remaining in the lungs at the end of a maximal expiration.

Resting heart rate (RHR) – The heart rate at resting levels measured in beats per minute (bpm).

Rheumatoid arthritis – Inflammatory disease of the joints.

RM – Repetition maximum.

Sarcomere – Unit of contraction in skeletal muscle.

Sarcoplasmic reticulum – System in skeletal muscle that releases calcium for muscle contraction.

Scoliosis – Twisting of the spine.

Screening – A process used to determine health status.

Serotonin – A compound that can induce vasoconstriction.

Sinoatrial node – The impulse-generating 'pacemaker' located in the right atrium.

Skill – Proficiency at a particular task.

Skinfolds – Indirect method of assessing body composition.

Slow twitch – Type of muscle fibre associated with endurance.

Smooth muscle – Muscle found in the walls of hollow organs that is not under voluntary control.

Speed – Movement per unit time with no particular direction.

Sphygmomanometer – A device that operates on barometric pressure in a mercury element used to measure blood pressure.

Spirometer – Device used to test lung function.

Stability – A body's resistance to the disturbance of equilibrium.

Stadiometer – Device used to measure height.

Stretch reflex – Reflex action causing contraction within a muscle.

Stretching – The method or technique used to influence the joint range of motion.

Stroke – A rapid disturbance to brain function lasting more than 24 hours.

Stroke volume – The amount of blood ejected from one ventricle per heartbeat.

Subcutaneous – A layer of tissue lying just below the dermis layer.

Supine – Lying on the back.

Sympathetic nervous system – Division of the autonomic nervous system, which can speed up the heart rate.

Synergist – A muscle or muscle group responsible for assisting the action.

Systolic – Maximum pressure on the artery walls during contraction of the left ventricle.

Tachycardia – High resting heart rate.

Telemetry – Method of remotely checking heart rate.

Tendon – Connective tissue that surrounds muscle fibres.

Testosterone – A hormone that is responsible for muscle growth.

Thermoregulation – The regulation of temperature using various systems within the body.

Tidal volume – The volume of air that is inhaled or exhaled with each breath.

Tissue – A collection of cells with a physiological function.

TLC – Total lung capacity.

Transversus abdominis – Muscle of the core involved in forced expiration.

Triglyceride – Type of fat used for fuel in the body.

Validity (test) – Purported to specifically measure what the tester or testing team is investigating.

Vasoconstriction – Narrowing of the lumen of blood vessels.

Vasodilation – Increase in size of lumen of blood vessels.

Vein – A vessel that caries blood back to the heart.

Velocity – Movement per unit time with direction.

Ventricle – A chamber in the heart that receives blood from the atrium.

Vestibular – Balance information sent to the brain as a result of the mechanism of the inner ear.

Viscosity – A measure of a fluid's resistance to flow.

VO$_2$ – Symbol for oxygen consumption.

VO$_2$max – Symbol for maximal oxygen consumption: the maximum amount of oxygen that can be delivered to the working muscles.

Voluntary – As a result of conscious thought.

Watts – A unit of power.

WHR – Waist-to-hip ratio.

INDEX